Chinese People's Time Use and Their Quality of Life

Fenglian Du · Wenbin Wang · Xiaoyuan Dong

Chinese People's Time Use and Their Quality of Life

Research Report of Chinese Time Use Survey

中国社会科学出版社
CHINA SOCIAL SCIENCES PRESS

Springer

Fenglian Du
School of Economics and Management
Inner Mongolia University
Hohhot, China

Wenbin Wang
China Time Use Survey and Research Center
Inner Mongolia University
Hohhot, China

Xiaoyuan Dong
Faculty of Business and Economics
The University of Winnipeg
Winnipeg, MB, Canada

Translated by
Yu Guan
School of Foreign Languages
University of Chinese Academy of Social Sciences
Beijing, China

ISBN 978-981-99-5525-1 ISBN 978-981-99-5526-8 (eBook)
https://doi.org/10.1007/978-981-99-5526-8

Jointly published with China Social Sciences Press
The print edition is not for sale in China (Mainland). Customers from China (Mainland) please order the print book from: China Social Sciences Press.
ISBN of the Co-Publisher's edition: 978-7-5203-2905-7

The work is supported by China Classics International.

Translation from the Chinese language edition: "《时间都去哪儿了?中国时间利用调查研究报告》" by Fenglian Du et al., © 2018. Published by China Social Sciences Press. All Rights Reserved.

This Springer imprint is published by the registered company Springer Nature Singapore Pte Ltd.
The registered company address is: 152 Beach Road, #21-01/04 Gateway East, Singapore 189721, Singapore

Contents

Part I
Tracing the Footsteps of Time: Survey Methods and Overview

Chapter 1
Survey Method

This chapter introduces the respondents, interview methods, survey contents, and sample distribution of the 2017 Chinese Time Use Survey (CTUS) based on a review of the history and the current status of the Global Time Use Survey (GTUS).

A Brief Introduction to the Time Use Survey

Every task a person undertakes requires a certain amount of time. Since the total amount of time that a person has each day is fixed, time is a very scarce and precious resource for everyone. The standard method for surveying people's time allocation is the Time Use Survey (TUS). The TUS is a quantitative measure of how individuals allocate their time to various activities in a given period (typically 24 h a day).[1]

It is a survey that has existed for nearly a century. As early as the 1920s, the Soviet Union and the United States had conducted Time Use Surveys.[2] The huge breakthrough of the TUS is the application of the Time Diary. In 1964, hosted by the Hungarian sociologist Alexander Szalai, 12 European countries joined forces to launch a multinational project that compared people's time budgets, which adopted an internationally comparable, Time Diary based survey method.[3] From then on, the Time Diary has been used as the fundamental survey method for the Global Time Use Survey.

[1] United Nations, *Guide to Producing Statistics on Time Use: Measuring Paid and Unpaid Work*, United Nations, Department of Economic and Social Affairs, Statistics Division, 2005, p. 5.

[2] Ironmonger D., "Time Use", *The New Palgrave Dictionary of Economics*, 2008.

[3] Szalai A. (Editor), *The Use of Time: Daily Activities of Urban and Suburban Populations in Twelve Countries*, The Hague: Mouton, 1972.

F. Du et al., *Chinese People's Time Use and Their Quality of Life*,
https://doi.org/10.1007/978-981-99-5526-8_1

In September 1995, the United Nations Fourth World Conference on Women was held in Beijing. The Beijing Declaration and Platform for Action, adopted at the conference, pointed out that women's low status in the family and society was due to the fact that much of their work was unpaid, and was neglected in the national economic accounting systems. Countries were called upon to "conduct regular TUS to quantify unpaid labor" in order to fully reflect women's contribution to the national economy and social welfare.[4] Since then, countries have been collecting and analyzing time use data on a large scale. The official and systematic TUS in the United States began in 2003 and is conducted annually by the Bureau of Labor Statistics of the United States Department of Labor. Worldwide, there are 65 countries that have conducted large-scale TUS.[5]

Since the 1980s, China has conducted Time Use Surveys in a few selected cities, such as Beijing.[6] In 2008, the first large-scale Time Use Survey in China was conducted by the National Bureau of Statistics. This survey was carried out in 10 provinces and cities, including Beijing, Hebei, Heilongjiang, Zhejiang, Anhui, Henan, Guangdong, Sichuan, Yunnan, and Gansu. The households' investigation was carried out in May of that year. A total of 37,142 household members aged 15–74 years from 16,661 households were investigated.[7]

In 2017, with the support of the National Program for Improving the Comprehensive Strength of Universities in Central and Western China, Inner Mongolia University joined the Research Data Sharing Platform of Universities in China and conducted a nationwide Time Use Survey in 29 provinces in the Chinese mainland, except Xinjiang and Tibet. The main survey was conducted from early July to early September of that year, with a follow-up phone call in October. The survey obtained time use information and related individual, family, and community information from 30,591 family members who were no younger than the age of 3, totaling 12,471 households. Given the seasonal nature of agricultural activities, in December of that year, the survey team interviewed members of the sample rural households by telephone about their time use during the slack season in farming.

Compared with the 2008 Time Use Survey of the National Bureau of Statistics of China, the 2017 Time Use Survey, although with a slightly smaller total sample size, has the following significant advances in methodology.

---

[4] United Nations, *Beijing Declaration and Platform for Action: Fourth World Conference on Women, Beijing, China*, United Nations Department of Policy Coordination and Sustainable Development, 1995.

[5] Charmes, Jacques, UNDP Human Development Report Office Background Paper: Time Use across the World: Findings of a World Compilation of Time Use Survey, 2015; Valeria Esquivel, Debbie Budlender, Nancy Folbre, et al., "Explorations: Time-use Surveys in the South", *Feminist Economics*, 2008, 14 (3): 107–152.

[6] Wei Yuan, Murakami Shokatsu, Qiyan Wang, A Comparative Study of Time Allocation of Beijing and Tokyo Residents, *Journal of Renmin University of China*, 2000 (03).

[7] Department of Social and Science and Technology Statistics, National Bureau of Statistics: *2008 Compilation of Time-use Surveys*, China Statistics Press, 2009 edition. In May 2018, NBS conducted another Time-use Survey in these 10 provinces, and the data from this survey have not yet been published.

(1) The number of provinces surveyed increased from 10 to 29, greatly enhancing the representativeness of the data for the whole country. (2) The age range of survey respondents was expanded from 15 to 74 years old to 3 years old and above, containing the study of the time use of young children and teenagers. (3) For respondents from the rural districts, the time use of their busy and slack season was obtained, allowing analysis of the seasonal changes in the time use of rural residents. (4) The classification of activities increased from 113 to 300, providing a more detailed depiction of human activities. (5) The 2017 Chinese Time Use Survey was conducted simultaneously with the China Household Finance Survey, and the samples of the former were part of the samples of the latter. Therefore, the 2017 Chinese Time Use Survey obtains extremely rich information on individuals, households, and communities in addition to time use data. The massive amount of information obtained by the 2017 Chinese Time Use Survey will make an important contribution to promoting time use research in China and filling the gaps in international time use research.

Respondents and Interview Methods

The respondents of the 2017 Chinese Time Use Survey (CTUS) were all household members not younger than 3 years old in urban and rural sample households in 29 provinces in Chinese mainland, except Xinjiang and Tibet. The sample households are about 12,000 households randomly selected from about 40,000 sample households of the 2017 China Household Finance Survey (CHFS). The survey is representative of the whole country and national urban and rural areas.

Each sample respondent filled out a Time Diary of a day. The survey obtained valid Time Diaries from a total of 30,591 respondents out of 12,471 urban and rural sample households, which were distributed in 1,417 communities nationwide, with a response rate of approximately 75%.

The main survey for the 2017 CTUS was conducted as a household visit from early July to early September. Interviewers were required to interview each member of the sample households in person as much as possible. When the respondents were under 12 years old or unfit to answer the questionnaire due to disability, illness, old age, etc., other members of the household could finish the interview on their behalves. For those household members who lived at their current address but could not be present for the interview and those who lived elsewhere (out for school, out for work, etc.), a computer-assisted telephone interview (CATI) was conducted in October. For respondents from the rural sample households, telephone interviews on their time use during the slack season in farming were conducted in December.

Survey Contents

Each survey respondent should complete a Time Diary featuring 24 h a day (from 4:00 a.m. the day before the household visit to 4:00 a.m. the same day) with the help of the interviewer, and with 10 min as the minimum time interval. The contents of the Time Diary are as follows.

As shown in Table 1.1, the Time Diary of the 2017 Chinese Time Use Survey contains five elements: (1) Who, (2) When, (3) What, (4) Where, and (5) With Whom.

(1) Who: The person who performs the activity.
(2) When: The time of a day when people engage in certain activities.
(3) What: The type of activity that people engage in. The survey divides all human activities into 11 divisions, 58 groups, and 300 sections; each division/group/section covers all human activities, and each division/group/section does not cross the other. The Time Diary collects not only major activities but also activities that are concurrent with the major activities. These activities are called secondary activities. There must be one and only one major activity for each time period, but the secondary activities are not necessary. If more than one secondary activity is engaged at the same time, only the most important secondary activity is to be taken into account. When engaging in multiple activities at the same time, it is up to the respondent to determine which activity is the major activity

Table 1.1 The time diary of the 2017 Chinese Time Use Survey

Time period	What are you doing? (Refers to the main activity being performed)	Where are you when engaged in the main activity? (Select the activity location code from the activity locations at the bottom of the table, or the transportation code if it is a transportation activity)	With whom are you while you are on your main activity? (Check the code for whom you are with. Multiple choices are allowed except for "alone")	What else are you doing at the same time? (Refers to secondary activities that you are doing at the same time as the main activity)	With whom are you doing the secondary activity? (Check the code for whom you are with. Multiple choices are allowed except for "alone")
4:00–4:10					
4:10–4:20					
4:20–4:30					
…					
…					
(To the next day)					

and which is the secondary one based on the major purpose of the activity. It is also necessary to record the time period of secondary activities, in the same way that major activities are recorded.

The list of 11 divisions of activities classified in this survey is shown in Table 1.2.

(4) Where: Where people's main activities take place. If the activity is other than transportation, fill in the location code; there are 14 divisions and 19 sections of the location code. If it is a transportation activity, fill in the transportation code; there are 11 divisions and 31 sections of the transportation code.

(5) With Whom: Who is with when engaging in major/secondary activities. The purpose of the activity serves as a basis for determining with whom to engage in major/secondary activities. Select the person code for certain activities. There are 9 divisions and 29 sections.

To obtain additional important information about the respondents, each household member was asked to answer 21 questions before filling out the Time Diary and 13 questions after it.

One question asked after filling out the Time Diary is whether the survey day is a typical day for the respondent in terms of time use. If the survey day is atypical, respondents must also be interviewed about their time use on a typical day. For workers, a typical day is a normal productive day or a normal day off (not working), while a holiday or a long vacation is atypical. For students, a typical day is a normal school day or a normal rest day (off school), while a holiday or a summer vacation is atypical.

Table 1.2 The divisions of activities classified in the 2017 Chinese Time Use Survey

Division code	Division name	Number of groups contained	Number of sections contained
01	Sleeping, personal hygiene activities, private activities	3	12
02	Eating and other dietary activities	2	6
03	Work and work-related activities	4	26
04	Getting educated	6	28
05	Home production and business activities	4	34
06	Doing household chores	9	19
07	Caring for family members and providing external help	6	37
08	Shopping, car repairs, haircuts, medical treatment, going to the bank, doing business, etc.	8	37
09	Physical exercise and fitness activities	5	24
10	Leisure and recreation	8	54
11	Social and religious activities	3	23

Sample Distribution

This section demonstrates the distribution of the 30,591 valid individual samples by gender, urban and rural division, ethnicity, age, week, education level, income, and province.

This survey uses weights to adjust for differences in sampling ratios and response rates across populations to ensure equal sample sizes across days of a week. Weights are used for all operations in this paper unless otherwise noted.

The gender and urban–rural distribution of the samples are shown in Tables 1.3 and 1.4. The results show that the weighted sample gender, urban–rural distribution, and overall national distribution are highly compatible.

The ethnic distribution of the sample is shown in Table 1.5. The results show that the proportion of minority ethnic groups in the weighted sample is slightly lower than the census number. The under-presence of samples from minority groups was caused by the fact that this survey did not cover the two minority autonomous regions of Xinjiang Uygur Autonomous Region and the Tibet Autonomous Region.

The age distributions of the samples are shown in Table 1.6 and Fig. 1.1. The results show that the age distribution of the weighted sample roughly matches the overall national distribution. The difference between the two is that compared with the overall distribution, there are slightly more samples from children, adolescents, and elderly people and slightly less working-age population in the Time Use Survey.

Table 1.3 Gender distribution of the 2017 Chinese Time Use Survey samples

Gender	Number of people	Unweighted sample percentage	Weighted sample percentage	Overall percentage[a]
Male	14,919	48.8	50.8	51.2
Female	15,672	51.2	49.2	48.8
Total	30,591	100	100	100

Note [a] The overall percentage is the year-end figure for 2017, and the data are obtained from the *Statistical Communiqué of the People's Republic of China on the 2017 National Economic and Social Development*, http://www.stats.gov.cn/tjsj/zxfb/201802/t20180228_1585631.html

Table 1.4 Urban–rural distribution of the 2017 Chinese Time Use Survey samples

Urban and rural	Individual sample size	Unweighted sample percentage	Weighted sample percentage	Overall percentage[a]
Urban	20,010	65.4	58.7	58.5
Rural	10,581	34.6	41.3	41.5
Total	30,591	100	100	100

Note [a] The overall percentage is the year-end figure for 2017, and the data are obtained from the *Statistical Communiqué of the People's Republic of China on the 2017 National Economic and Social Development*, http://www.stats.gov.cn/tjsj/zxfb/201802/t20180228_1585631.html

Table 1.5 Ethnic distribution of the 2017 Chinese Time Use Survey samples

Urban and rural	Individual sample size	Unweighted sample percentage	Weighted sample percentage	Overall percentage[b]
The Han nationality	28,240	92.3	92.2	91.5
Ethnic minorities	2350	7.7	7.8	8.5
Total	30,590[a]	100	100	100

Note [a] There is one person in the sample with unknown ethnicity; [b] This is the 1% national sample census in 2015. The data is from *The 2015 National 1% Population Sample Census*

Table 1.6 Age distribution of the 2017 Chinese Time Use Survey samples

Age	Number of people	Unweighted sample percentage	Weighted sample percentage	Overall percentage[a]
3–15 year old	3822	12.0.5	16.9	14.7
16–50 year old	16,919	55.3	64.7	68.6
60 years and older	9850	32.2	18.4	16.7
Total	30,591	100	100	100

Note [a] The Overall Percentage represents the 1% national sample census in 2015. The data is from *The 2015 National 1% Population Sample Census*

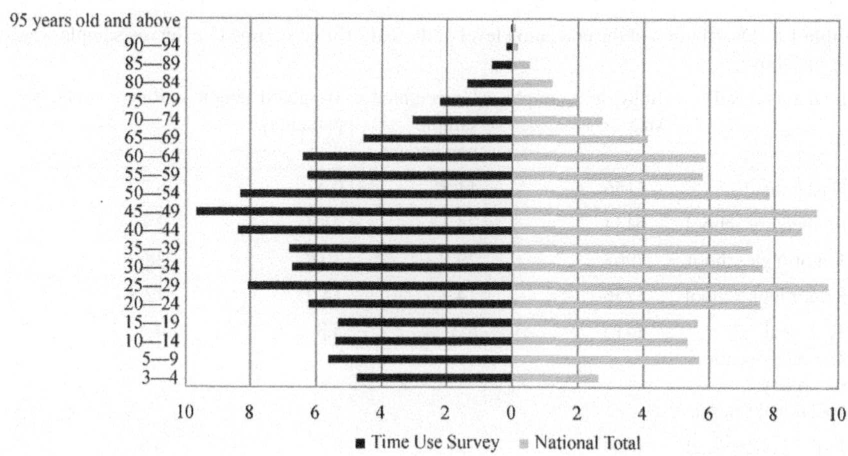

Fig. 1.1 Age structure of the 2017 Chinese Time Use Survey

The weekly distribution is shown in Table 1.7. The results show that the weighted sample week distribution roughly matches the natural distribution (1/7 of the day).

The distribution of education levels of the samples is shown in Table 1.8. Since only respondents aged 16 and above were asked about their education levels in the survey, the distribution of this part of the samples is presented here. The results show that the weighted distribution of the sample's education levels roughly matches the overall national distribution.

The income distribution of the samples is shown in Table 1.9, which is in decile groups based on national per capita household income. The results show that the

Table 1.7 Weekly distribution of the 2017 Chinese Time Use Survey samples

Days of a week	Individual sample size	Unweighted sample percentage	Weighted sample percentage	Raw percentage
Monday	4772	15.6	14.7	14.3
Tuesday	4792	15.7	14.6	14.3
Wednesday	4674	15.3	14.8	14.3
Thursday	4547	14.9	15.1	14.3
Friday	4468	14.6	15.6	14.3
Saturday	3352	11.0	12.4	14.3
Sunday	3986	13.0	12.9	14.3
Total	30,591	100	100	100

Table 1.8 Distribution of the education level of the 2017 Chinese Time Use Survey samples (aged 16 and above)

Education level	Individual sample size	Unweighted sample percentage	Weighted sample percentage	Raw percentage[a]
Unschooled	3156	11.8	9.4	5.7
Elementary school	6434	24.1	21.4	25.6
Junior high school	7963	29.8	30.8	38.8
Senior high school	3756	14.1	14.2	12.8
Technical secondary school/ secondary vocational school	1416	5.3	5.8	4.2
Junior college/high vocational school	1864	7.0	8.1	6.9
Undergraduate	1947	7.3	9.5	5.5
Graduate	171	0.6	0.8	0.5
Total	26,709	100	100	100

Note [a] The overall percentage is the percentage of the education levels of the population aged 6 and above in 2016. The data is from *China Statistical Yearbook 2017*

Table 1.9 Income distribution of the 2017 Chinese Time Use Survey samples

Decile groups	Lowest income	Highest income	Weighted number	Per capita income	Weighted percentage
1	–	1592	3059	−1593	10.0
2	1592	4359	3059	2979	10.0
3	4359	7232	3058	5862	10.0
4	7232	10,362	3055	8705	10.0
5	10,362	13,940	3064	12,099	10.0
6	13,940	18,616	3057	16,199	10.0
7	18,616	24,683	3061	21,410	10.0
8	24,683	33,800	3059	28,817	10.0
9	33,800	51,258	3056	41,135	10.0
10	51,258	–	3063	113,359	10.0
Total	–	–	30,591	24,908	100.0

median annual per capita income was RMB 13,940 per person, which is significantly lower than the mean value of RMB 24,908 per person. Compared with the national per capita disposable income of RMB 25,974 and the median of RMB 22,408 in 2017,[8] the mean income roughly matches the mean value, and the median income is significantly lower. This implies that the majority of the respondents' self-reported income is low.

Finally, Table 1.10 presents the distribution of this survey sample across provinces, which is the unweighted sample distribution.

Summary

The Time Use Survey uses the method of filling out Time Diaries to collect information on what activities individuals engage in during a specific period (generally a day) and how much time is spent on each activity and is a standard method for investigating people's time resource allocation. This chapter introduces the respondents, interview method, survey content, and sample distribution of the 2017 Chinese Time Use Survey (CTUS).

The 2017 Chinese Time Use Survey was jointly conducted by the Inner Mongolia University and the Southwest University of Finance and Economics. The survey samples are consisted of more or less 12,000 households randomly selected from about 40,000 sample households in the 2017 China Household Financial Survey (CHFS). The survey collected valid Time Diaries from 30,591 respondents in 29 provinces in Chinese mainland, except Xinjiang and Tibet, and is representative of

[8] *Statistical Communiqué of the People's Republic of China on the 2017 National Economic and Social Development.*

Table 1.10 Province distribution of the 2017 Chinese Time Use Survey samples

Provinces	Individual sample size
Anhui province	913
Beijing municipality	843
Fujian province	1247
Gansu province	713
Guangdong province	1783
Guangxi Zhuang autonomous region	808
Guizhou province	687
Hainan province	916
Hebei province	1440
Henan province	1140
Heilongjiang province	832
Hubei province	937
Hunan province	1297
Jilin province	1019
Jiangsu province	1417
Jiangxi province	782
Liaoning province	997
Inner Mongolia autonomous region	1117
Ningxia Hui autonomous region	477
Qinghai province	699
Shandong province	1187
Shanxi province	1236
Shaanxi province	720
Shanghai municipality	1598
Sichuan province	1353
Tianjin municipality	865
Yunnan province	968
Zhejiang province	1350
Chongqing municipality	1250
Total	30,591

the whole country, including urban and rural areas, with a response rate of about 75%. The survey system collects information on four aspects of when people engage in what types of activities, where they engage in these activities, and who they are with when they engage in these activities.

The distributions of the individual sample by gender, urban/rural, ethnicity, age, and education level match the overall national sample fairly well.

Chapter 2
Time Use Overview

The 2017 Chinese Time Use Survey has obtained detailed data on the time allocation of Chinese residents. Based on these data, the first section of this chapter presents a basic overview of the time use of Chinese residents in 2017, comparing the time use of different genders, urban and rural areas, ages, and education levels.

From 2008 to 2017, China's total economic volume, industrial structure, and urbanization have all undergone significant changes. Accordingly, people's time use also changes. The second section of this chapter analyzes the evolution of the time allocation of Chinese residents based on the only two sets of large-scale Time Use Survey data available in China (conducted in 2008 and 2017, respectively).

Because countries are at different development stages and have different cultural backgrounds, time use also differs. The third section of this chapter compares the differences of time use between China and 10 major developed countries, as well as four developing countries and transitional countries, based on comparable international Time Use Survey data.

The analysis in this chapter divides human activities into five categories: paid labor, unpaid labor, studying and training, leisure and social activities, and self-care. Each category of activity is defined as shown in Table 2.1.

Overview of Time Use of Chinese Residents in 2017

Basic Information

Based on data from the 2017 Chinese Time Use Survey, this subsection describes the time use of Chinese residents aged 3 years and above, as well as the differences in time use by gender and by urban and rural division.

The average participation length of various activities, participation rate, and average participant duration of Chinese residents are shown in Table 2.2 and Fig. 2.1.

F. Du et al., *Chinese People's Time Use and Their Quality of Life*,
https://doi.org/10.1007/978-981-99-5526-8_2

Table 2.1 Activities

Activity name	Divisions of activities included
Paid labor	03 Work and work-related activities
	05 Household production and management activities
Unpaid labor	06 Doing housework
	07 Taking care of family members and providing assistance to the outside world
	08 Shopping, car repair, haircut, medical treatment, going to the bank, doing business, etc.
Education and training	04 Getting educated
Leisure and social activities	09 Physical exercise and fitness activities
	10 Recreation and leisure
	11 Social interaction and religious activities
Self-care	01 Sleeping, personal hygiene activities, and private activities
	02 Eating and other dietary activities

Table 2.2 Basic information about each type of activity

Activity	Average hours per day	Participation rate (%)	Participants' average hours per day
Paid labor	4.16	49.9	8.34
Unpaid labor	1.84	50.8	3.62
Studying and training	1.48	17.5	8.49
Leisure and social activities	4.63	88.4	5.24
Self-care	11.88	100.0	11.88

It can be found that, as the main way to obtain income, Chinese residents' paid labor time was 4.16 h per day; half of the residents performed paid labor on the survey day. Unpaid labor occupied 1.84 h per day; slightly more than half of the residents performed unpaid labor on the survey day. Total labor (the sum of paid and unpaid labor) was 6.00 h per day, accounting for a quarter of a whole day.

Chinese residents spent 1.48 h per day on studying and training; slightly more than 1/6 of the residents on the survey day were engaged in studying and training, and the majority were students. Leisure and social activities took 4.63 h per day; only 1/9 of the residents did not do any leisure or social activities on the survey day. The average length of self-care was 11.88 h per day, almost half of a whole day; the participation rate in self-care was 100%. After all, almost no one sleeps or eats throughout the day.

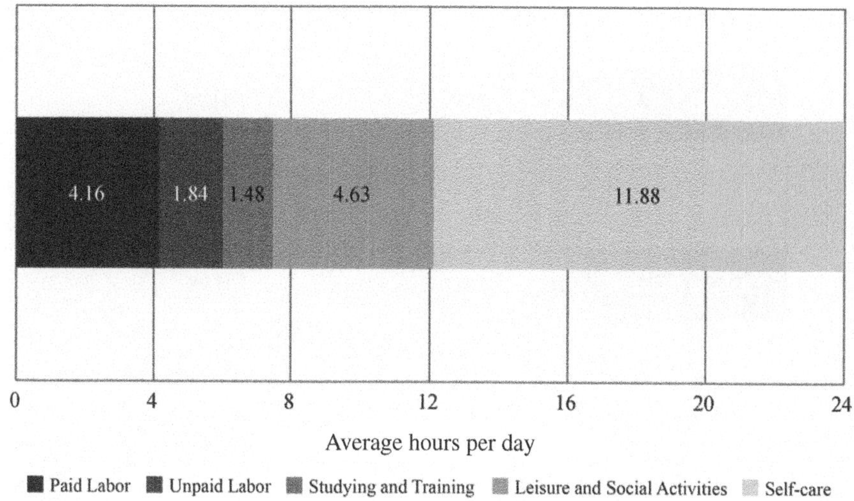

Fig. 2.1 The average length of various types of activities

The average participation length of various activities, participation rate, and average participant duration for Chinese male and female residents are shown in Table 2.3 and Fig. 2.2.

It can be found that there are gender differences in all five types of activities, especially in paid and unpaid labor, showing a clear pattern of "men's work centers around outside, while women's work centers around home". Men's paid labor time was 1.42 h higher than women's per day; men's paid labor participation rate was 12% points higher than that of women. However, women's unpaid labor time was 1.85 h higher than men's per day, which was three times higher than the latter's; women's unpaid labor participation rate was 32.1% points higher than that of men. The total labor time (sum of paid and unpaid labor) of women was 0.43 h higher than that of men per day.

Table 2.3 Gender differences in various types of activities

Activity	Average hours per day		Participation rate (%)		Participants' average hours per day	
	Male	Female	Male	Female	Male	Female
Paid labor	4.86	3.44	55.8	43.8	8.72	7.85
Unpaid labor	0.93	2.78	35.0	67.1	2.65	4.15
Studying and training	1.58	1.38	18.5	16.4	8.55	8.43
Leisure and social activities	4.85	4.41	90.1	86.6	5.39	5.09
Self-care	11.78	11.98	100	100	11.78	11.98

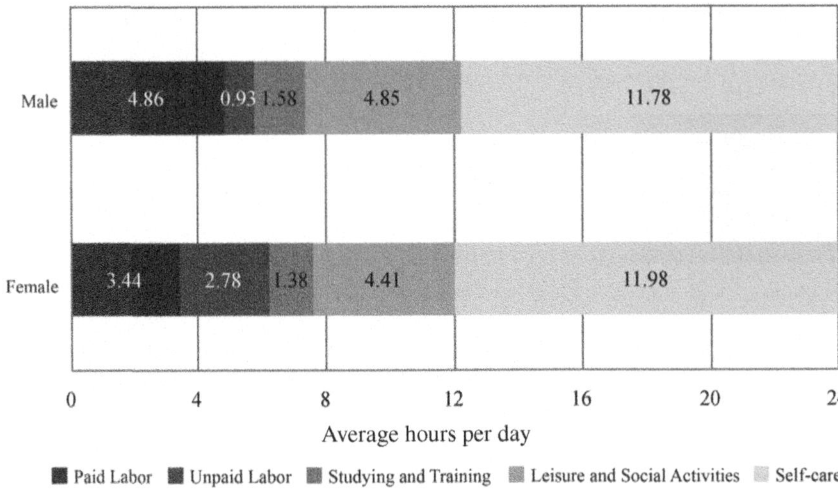

Fig. 2.2 Gentler differences in the average participation length of each type of activity

The average participation length and participation rates of studying and training, leisure and social activities were slightly higher for men than for women. Women spent slightly more time on self-care than men.

The average participation length of various activities, participation rate, and average participant duration of urban and rural residents in China are shown in Table 2.4 and Fig. 2.3.

It can be found that the urban–rural differences in the five types of activities are not very significant. The paid labor, unpaid labor, and total labor time (the sum of paid and unpaid labor) of rural residents were all slightly higher than those of urban residents. The participation rate of paid labor was significantly higher for rural residents than for urban residents, while the participation length of paid labor was significantly higher for urban residents than for rural residents.

Table 2.4 Urban–rural differences in various types of activities

Activity	Average hours per day		Participation rate (%)		Participants' average hours per day	
	Urban	Rural	Urban	Rural	Urban	Rural
Paid labor	4.13	4.21	47.1	53.9	8.77	7.80
Unpaid labor	1.80	1.90	50.8	50.9	3.55	3.74
Studying and training	1.55	1.39	18.3	16.3	8.48	8.51
Leisure and social activities	4.71	4.52	89.0	87.5	5.30	5.17
Self-care	11.80	11.98	100	100	11.80	11.98

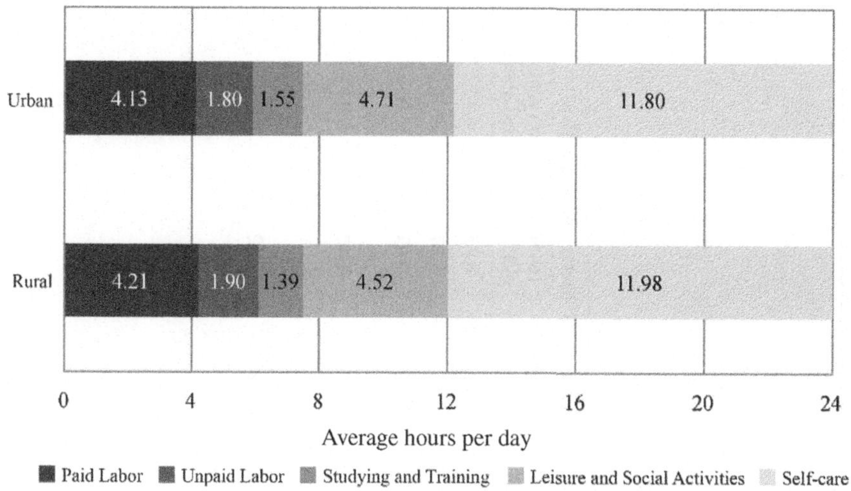

Fig. 2.3 Urban–rural differences in the average participation length of each type of activity

The average hours of studying and training and the participation rate in leisure and social activities were slightly higher for urban residents than for rural residents. The self-care time of rural residents was slightly higher than that of urban residents.

Time Use of Residents of Different Ages

This subsection analyzes the time use of residents of different ages in China in 2017, as well as gender and urban–rural differences in the time use of residents in different age groups.

According to China's division of pre-labor, labor, and post-labor ages, residents were divided into three age groups: 3–15 years old, 16–59 years old, and 60 years old and above, which corresponded to children and adolescents, middle-aged and young adults, and older adults, respectively. Among the total samples, the percentages of residents in these three age groups were 17%, 65%, and 18%, respectively.

The time use of residents of different ages is shown in Table 2.5 and Fig. 2.4.

It can be found that the average participation length of the five types of activities changed very regularly at different stages of life. Paid labor time was close to none for children and adolescents, jumped to nearly 6 h per day for middle-aged and young adults, and halved as people entered old age. Unpaid labor time was close to none for children and adolescents, jumped to more than 2 h per day for middle-aged and young adults, and continued to increase when people enter old age. Studying and training time was mainly concentrated in the school-age group, i.e., children and adolescents, as well as in the early middle-aged and young adults. Leisure and social

Table 2.5 Time use of residents of different ages

Activity	Average hours per day			Participation rate (%)			Participants' average hours per day		
	3–15 years old	16–50 years old	60 years old and above	3–15 years old	16–50 years old	60 years old and above	3–15 years old	16–50 years old	60 years old and above
Paid labor	0.12	5.74	2.34	4.3	65.7	36.3	2.85	8.73	6.45
Unpaid labor	0.14	2.06	2.63	8.7	56.2	70.6	1.67	3.67	3.73
Studying and training	5.86	0.76	0.03	70.4	8.4	0.9	8.32	9.03	2.91
Leisure and social activities	4.99	3.93	6.78	91.0	86.0	94.1	5.49	4.57	7.21
Self-care	12.88	11.52	12.22	100	100	100	12.88	11.52	12.22

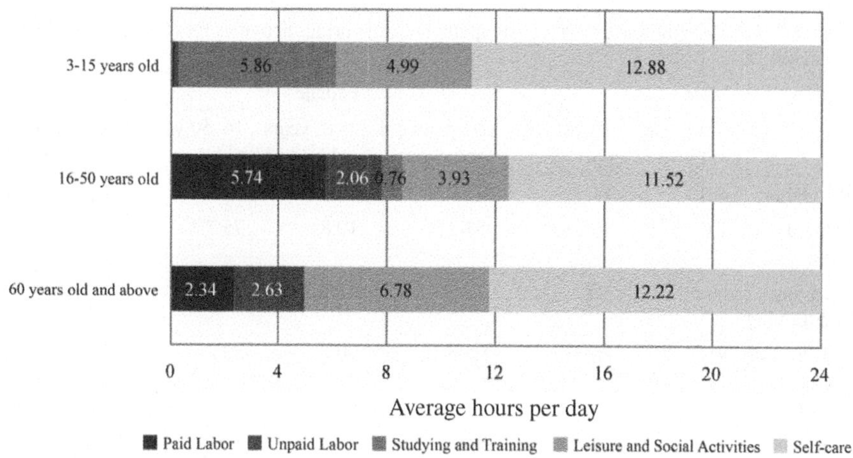

Fig. 2.4 Average participation length of various activities for residents of different ages

time decreased and then increased with age. Self-care time varied less significantly with age but also decreased and then increased as people grew.

The gender differences in time use of residents of different ages are shown in Tables 2.6 and 2.7, and Fig. 2.5.

It can be found that the average participation length of the five types of activities varied in a very similar pattern with age for men and women. The gender differences were mainly reflected in the fact that the unpaid labor time of women increased slightly at a high level while that of men increased significantly at a low level as people grew from middle age to old age.

The urban–rural differences in the time use of residents of different ages are shown in Tables 2.8 and 2.9, and Fig. 2.6.

Table 2.6 Gender differences in the average participation length of various activities for residents of different ages. Unit: hours/day

Activity	Male			Female		
	3–15 years old	16–50 years old	60 years old and above	3–15 years old	16–50 years old	60 years old and above
Paid labor	0.12	6.77	2.90	0.12	4.70	1.81
Unpaid labor	0.13	0.93	1.75	0.16	3.20	3.46
Studying and training	5.87	0.78	0.02	5.86	0.73	0.03
Leisure and social activities	5.09	4.15	7.14	4.88	3.70	6.44
Self-care	12.80	11.38	12.17	12.98	11.66	12.26

Table 2.7 Gender differences in the participation rate of various activities for residents of different ages. Unit: %

Activity	Male			Female		
	3–15 years old	16–50 years old	60 years old and above	3–15 years old	16–50 years old	60 years old and above
Paid labor	4.6	74.3	42.0	3.9	57.0	30.9
Unpaid labor	7.0	36.9	57.3	10.8	75.7	83.2
Studying and training	69.9	8.5	1.1	71.0	8.2	0.7
Leisure and social activities	91.3	88.3	95.3	90.7	83.7	93.1
Self-care	100	100	100	100	100	100

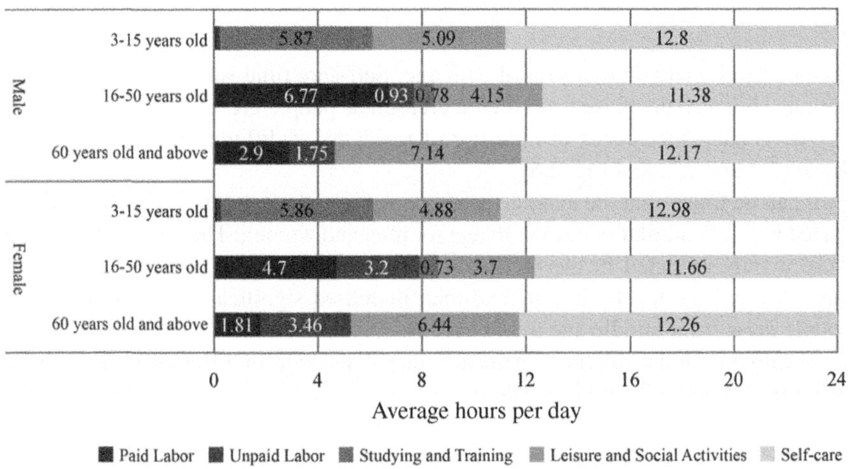

Fig. 2.5 Gender differences in the average participation length of various activities for residents of different ages

It can be found that the average participation length of the five types of activities of urban and rural residents changed in a similar pattern with age. The urban–rural differences were mainly reflected in that when growing from middle age to old age, the paid labor time declined significantly for urban residents, but was distinctly less significant for rural residents; the unpaid labor time increased significantly for urban residents, while only slightly for rural residents; and the increase in leisure and social time increased significantly for urban residents, while the increase was significantly lower for rural residents.

Table 2.8 Urban–rural differences in the average participation length of various activities for residents of different ages. Unit: hours/day

Activity	Urban			Rural		
	3–15 years old	16–50 years old	60 years old and above	3–15 years old	16–50 years old	60 years old and above
Paid labor	0.09	5.83	1.58	0.16	5.59	3.32
Unpaid labor	0.13	1.95	2.82	0.16	2.23	2.38
Studying and training	6.24	0.77	0.04	5.35	0.73	0.01
Leisure and social activities	4.64	4.00	7.44	5.46	3.82	5.95
Self-care	12.89	11.44	12.12	12.86	11.63	12.34

Table 2.9 Urban–rural differences in the participation rate of various activities for residents of different ages. Unit: %

Activity	Urban			Rural		
	3–15 years old	16–50 years old	60 years old and above	3–15 years old	16–50 years old	60 years old and above
Paid labor	3.2	64.9	22.0	5.7	66.9	54.6
Unpaid labor	7.4	55.8	72.9	10.4	56.8	67.7
Studying and training	74.7	8.6	1.1	64.6	7.9	0.6
Leisure and social activities	89.7	87.0	95.5	92.7	84.5	92.4
Self-care	100	100	100	100	100	100

Time Use of Residents with Different Education Levels

This subsection analyzes the time use of residents with different education levels in China in 2017, as well as the gender and urban–rural differences in the time use of residents with different education levels. Since information on education level is only available for the samples aged 16 and above, this subsection analyzes residents aged 16 and above.

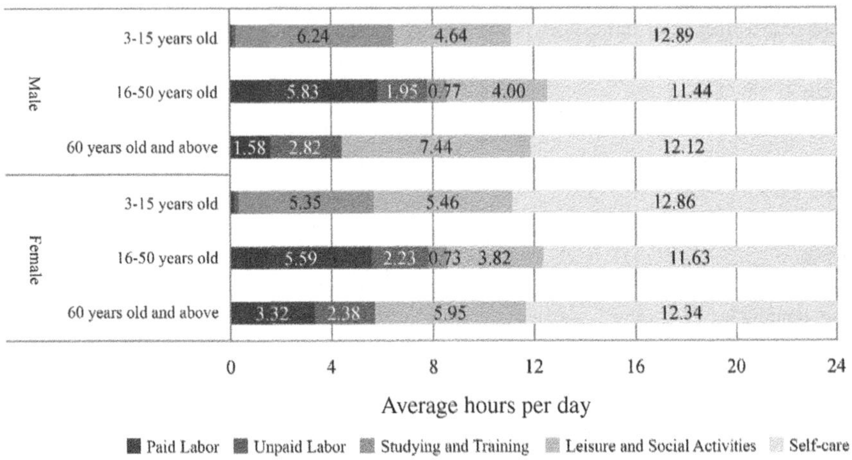

Fig. 2.6 Urban–rural differences in the average participation length of various activities for residents of different ages

Based on the education level, residents were divided into four groups: elementary school and below, junior high school, senior high school or secondary vocational high school, and college and above. Among the total sample, the percentages of residents in these four groups of different education levels were 31%, 31%, 20%, and 18%, respectively.

The time use of residents with different education levels is shown in Table 2.10 and Fig. 2.7.

It can be found that the average participation length of the five types of activities varied with the residents' education level, and this variation shows a certain pattern. As residents' education level improved, the change of paid labor time became irregular, the unpaid labor time decreased, the study and training time rose before it fell (which mainly reflects the difference in the proportion of students in each population), the leisure and social time decreased, and the self-care time first fell and then rose.

The gender differences in time use of residents with different education levels are shown in Tables 2.11 and 2.12, and Fig. 2.8.

It can be found that the average participation length of the five types of activities varied similarly with the education level for both men and women. However, it is noteworthy that the difference in unpaid labor time between men and women narrowed significantly as the education level increased.

Table 2.10 Time use of residents by education levels (of the population aged 16 years and above)

Activity	Average hours per day				Participation rate (%)				Participants' average hours per day			
	Elementary school and below	Junior high school	Senior high school or secondary vocational high school	College and above	Elementary school and below	Junior high school	Senior high school or secondary vocational high school	College and above	Elementary school and below	Junior high school	Senior high school or secondary vocational high school	College and above
Paid labor	4.43	5.56	4.55	5.46	57.6	63.0	52.7	62.8	7.68	8.82	8.63	8.70
Unpaid labor	2.61	2.27	1.97	1.57	68.1	60.3	53.2	50.1	3.83	3.76	3.71	3.14
Studying and training	0.04	0.23	1.55	1.09	0.7	2.8	14.8	14.4	4.96	8.17	10.47	7.60
Leisure and social activities	5.05	4.44	4.39	4.12	88.0	87.7	86.8	88.9	5.74	5.07	5.05	4.63
Self-care	11.88	11.50	11.54	11.76	100	100	100	100	11.88	11.50	11.54	11.76

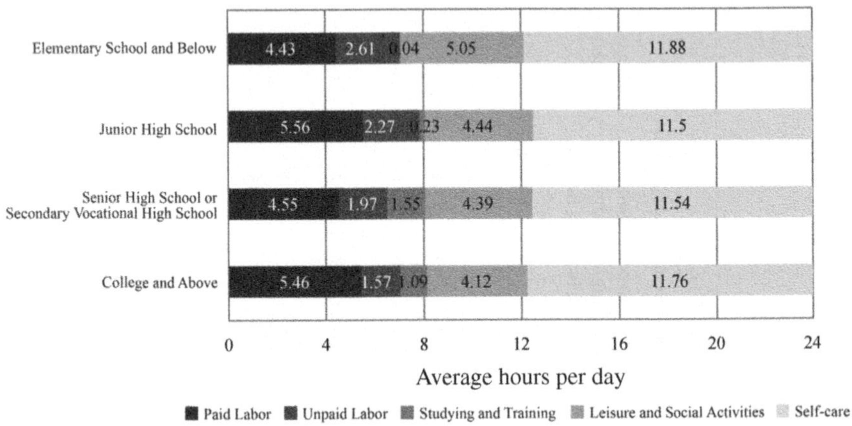

Fig. 2.7 Average participation length of various activities for residents with different education levels

Table 2.11 Gender differences in the average participation length of various activities for residents with different education levels (of the population aged 16 and above). Unit: hours/day

Activity	Male				Female			
	Elementary school and below	Junior high school	Senior high school or secondary vocational high school	College and above	Elementary school and below	Junior high school	Senior high school or secondary vocational high school	College and above
Paid labor	5.59	6.47	5.46	5.97	3.67	4.47	3.45	4.85
Unpaid labor	1.23	1.13	1.04	0.98	3.51	3.62	3.09	2.28
Studying and training	0.04	0.23	1.45	1.06	0.03	0.24	1.68	1.14
Leisure and social activities	5.31	4.72	4.65	4.45	4.88	4.11	4.07	3.72
Self-care	11.83	11.44	11.40	11.54	11.91	11.57	11.71	12.02

The urban–rural differences in the time use of residents with different education levels are shown in Tables 2.13 and 2.14 and Fig. 2.9.

Table 2.12 Gender differences in the participation rate of various activities for residents with different education levels (of the population aged 16 and above). Unit: %

Activity	Male				Female			
	Elementary school and below	Junior high school	Senior high school or secondary vocational high school	College and above	Elementary school and below	Junior high school	Senior high school or secondary vocational high school	College and above
Paid labor	66.3	71.1	62.3	67.9	52.0	53.4	41.0	56.6
Unpaid labor	44.4	41.1	38.4	40.6	83.5	82.9	70.9	61.6
Studying and training	0.9	2.5	14.0	13.7	0.6	3.0.2	15.8	15.2
Leisure and social activities	88.2	90.0	90.1	91.0	87.8	85.0	82.9	86.3
Self-care	100	100	100	100	100	100	100	100

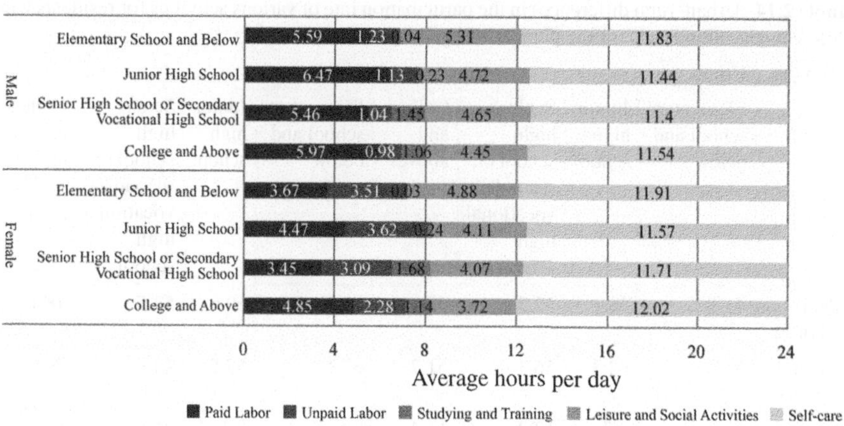

Fig. 2.8 Gender differences in the average participation length of various activities for residents with different education levels (of the population aged 16 and above)

It can be found that the average participation length of the five types of activities for urban and rural residents changed similarly with the education level. However, it is noteworthy that the differences in leisure and social activities between urban and rural residents narrowed significantly as the education level increased.

Table 2.13 Urban–rural differences in the average participation length of various activities for residents with different education levels (of the population aged 16 and above). Unit: hours/day

Activity	Urban				Rural			
	Elementary school and below	Junior high school	Senior high school or secondary vocational high school	College and above	Elementary school and below	Junior high school	Senior high school or secondary vocational high school	College and above
Paid labor	3.57	5.35	4.66	5.68	4.90	5.83	4.25	4.06
Unpaid labor	2.77	2.27	2.04	1.61	2.52	2.26	1.80	1.28
Studying and training	0.06	0.20	1.29	0.86	0.02	0.28	2.21	2.56
Leisure and social activities	5.71	4.76	4.58	4.13	4.68	4.02	3.90	4.02
Self-care	11.88	11.42	11.43	11.71	11.87	11.61	11.84	12.08

Table 2.14 Urban–rural differences in the participation rate of various activities for residents with different education levels (of the population aged 16 and above). Unit: %

Activity	Urban				Rural			
	Elementary school and below	Junior high school	Senior high school or secondary vocational high school	College and above	Elementary school and below	Junior high school	Senior high school or secondary vocational high school	College and above
Paid labor	43.1	58.1	52.7	65.1	65.7	69.6	52.5	48.1
Unpaid labor	69.8	62.3	56.4	51.7	67.1	57.8	44.9	39.6
Studying and training	1.1	2.7	12.2	11.4	0.5	3.1	21.5	33.5
Leisure and social activities	90.0	88.8	88.0	88.8	86.9	86.2	84.0	89.7
Self-care	100	100	100	100	100	100	100	100

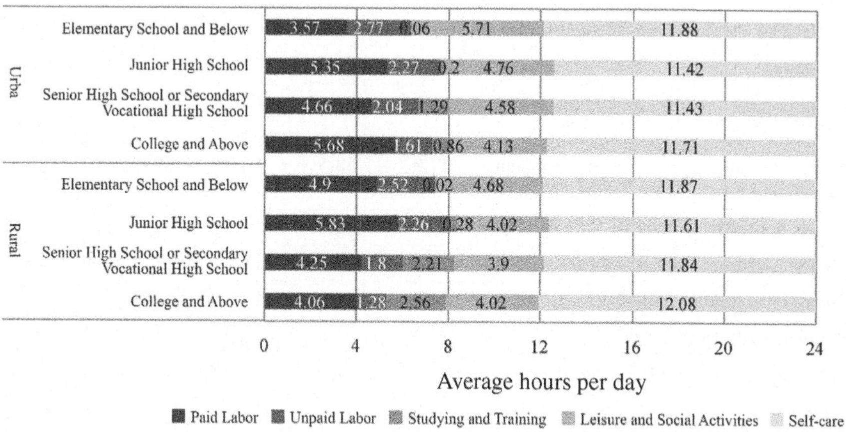

Fig. 2.9 Urban–rural differences in the average participation length of various activities for residents with different education levels

Changes in the Time Use of Chinese Residents from 2008 to 2017

From 2008 to 2017, China's economic and social conditions have undergone significant changes. The total economic volume has doubled, the share of output and employment in the tertiary sector has increased significantly, the share of employment in the primary industry has dropped sharply, and the urbanization rate has rocketed. The relevant main indicators are shown in Table 2.15.

Economic development and social changes are inevitably reflected in the time use of residents. This section compares the time use of Chinese residents in 2008 and 2017 based on the only two sets of large-scale Time Use Survey data available in China.

The National Bureau of Statistics conducted the first Chinese large-scale Time Use Survey in 2008 and published a compilation of the data in the following year.[1] Since the 2008 survey was conducted among the population aged 15–74 in the surveyed households, this section calculates the time use of the sample aged 15–74 in the 2017 survey for comparability of different age groups.

The 2008 survey covered 10 provinces and one municipality, namely the Beijing Municipality, Hebei, Heilongjiang, Zhejiang, Anhui, Henan, Guangdong, Sichuan, Yunnan, and Gansu (the survey provinces were selected considering the representativeness of geography and economic development), while the 2017 survey covered 29 provinces (all other provinces of Chinese mainland except Xinjiang and Xizang). To determine the impact of the change in the geographic scope of the survey on the

[1] Department of Social and Science and Technology Statistics, National Bureau of Statistics: *2008 Compilation of Time-use Survey Information*, China Statistics Press, 2009 edition. In May 2018, NBS conducted another Time-use Survey in these 10 provinces, and the data from this survey have not yet been published.

Table 2.15 Major economic and social development indicators in China from 2008 to 2017

Indicator	2008	2017	Changes from 2008 to 2017
Total population at the end of the year (billion people)	13.28	13.90	Up by 4.7%
Urbanization rate of permanent residents population (%)	47.0	58.5	Up by 11.5% points
Gross domestic product (trillion Yuan)	31.95	82.71	Up by 102% in real terms
Share of primary industry (%)	10.3	7.9	Down by 2.4% points
Share of secondary industry (%)	46.9	40.5	Down by 6.4% points
Share of tertiary industry (%)	42.8	51.6	Up by 8.8% points
Per capita GDP (Yuan)	24,121	59,660	Up by 93% in real terms
Employed population (billion people)	7.56	7.76	Up by 2.6%
Share of primary industry (%)	39.6	27.7[a]	Down by 11.9% points
Share of secondary industry (%)	27.2	28.8[a]	Up by 1.6% points
Share of tertiary industry (%)	33.2	43.5[a]	Up by 10.3% points

Note [a] Data in 2016
Source National Bureau of Statistics, http://data.stats.gov.cn/easyquery.htm?cn=C01; *Statistical Communiqué of the People's Republic of China on the 2017 National Economic and Social Development*, http://www.stats.gov.cn/tjsj/zxfb/201802/t20180228_1585631.html

survey results, Table 2.16 and Fig. 2.10 compare the average participation length of each type of activity in the 10 provinces in 2017 (the exact same provinces as the 2008 survey) with those in the 29 provinces.

As presented, there is a non-negligible difference between the 10-province results and the 29-province results in 2017. Therefore, this chapter adopts the 10-province data in 2017 to compare with the 2008s to exclude the effect of changes in the survey range.

Table 2.16 Comparison of the average participation length of various types of activities for the two geographic ranges in 2017. Unit: hours/day

Range	Activity	Total	Male	Female	Urban	Rural
10 Provinces	Paid labor	5.26	6.22	4.31	5.23	5.30
	Unpaid labor	2.17	1.04	3.28	2.12	2.22
	Studying and training	0.78	0.79	0.76	0.82	0.73
	Leisure and social activities	4.08	4.33	3.84	4.22	3.93
	Self-care	11.71	11.62	11.81	11.61	11.82
29 Provinces	Paid labor	5.15	6.09	4.20	5.11	5.20
	Unpaid labor	2.18	1.08	3.30	2.11	2.28
	Studying and training	0.74	0.77	0.70	0.77	0.69
	Leisure and social activities	4.34	4.58	4.09	4.50	4.12
	Self-care	11.60	11.48	11.71	11.52	11.71

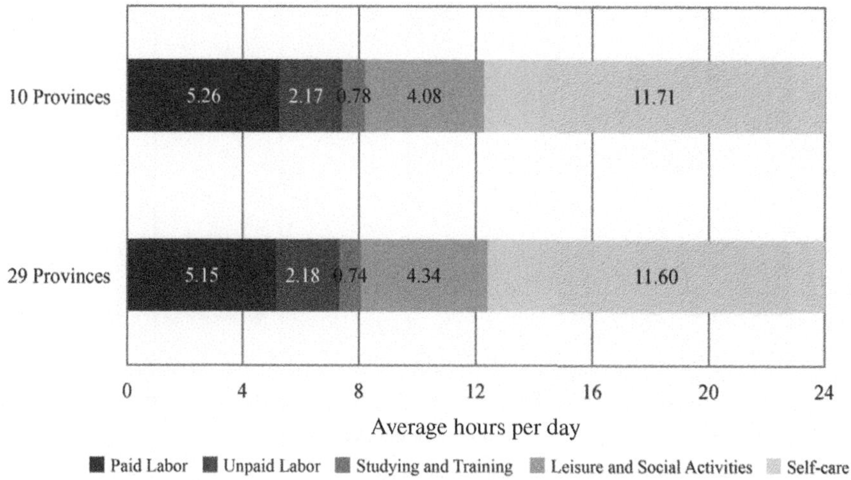

Fig. 2.10 Comparison of the average participation length of various types of activities in 10 provinces and 29 provinces in 2017

Overview

From 2008 to 2017, the changes in the time use of Chinese residents are shown in Table 2.17, Figs. 2.11, 2.12, and 2.13.

The pattern of time use of Chinese adults has changed significantly from 2008 to 2017. Paid labor time increased slightly. Unpaid labor time decreased by 0.55 h per day, which may be related to the outsourcing of some household chores, the popularity of time-saving household appliances, and the rise of online shopping. Total work (paid labor + unpaid labor) time decreased by 0.47 h per day. Studying

Table 2.17 Comparison of the average participation length of various types of activities between 2008 and 2017. Unit: hours/day

Year	Activity	Total	Male	Female	Urban	Rural
2008	Paid labor	5.18	6.00	4.38	4.12	6.35
	Unpaid labor	2.72	1.50	3.90	2.93	2.50
	Studying and training	0.55	0.57	0.52	0.63	0.45
	Leisure and social activities	3.90	4.22	3.60	4.63	3.12
	Self-care	11.63	11.70	11.58	11.68	11.57
2017	Paid labor	5.26	6.22	4.31	5.23	5.30
	Labor	2.17	1.04	3.28	2.12	2.22
	Studying and training	0.78	0.79	0.76	0.82	0.73
	Leisure and social activities	4.08	4.33	3.84	4.22	3.93
	Self-care	11.71	11.62	11.81	11.61	11.82

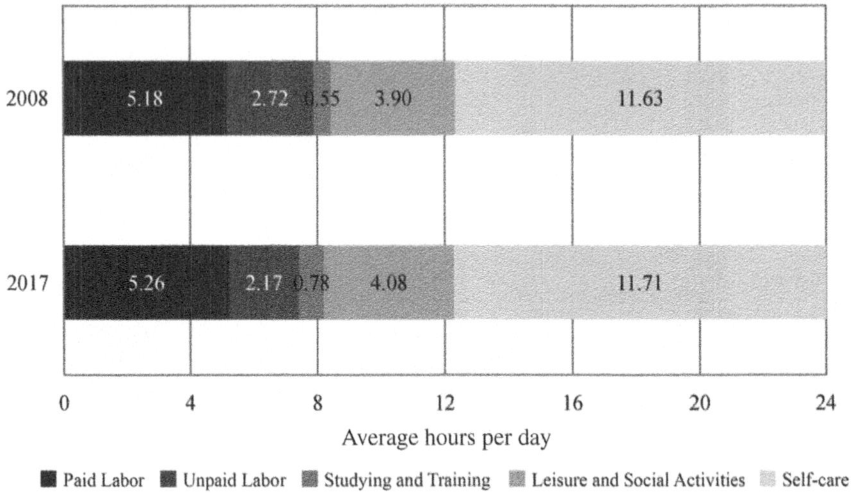

Fig. 2.11 Comparison of the average participation length of various types of activities between 2008 and 2017

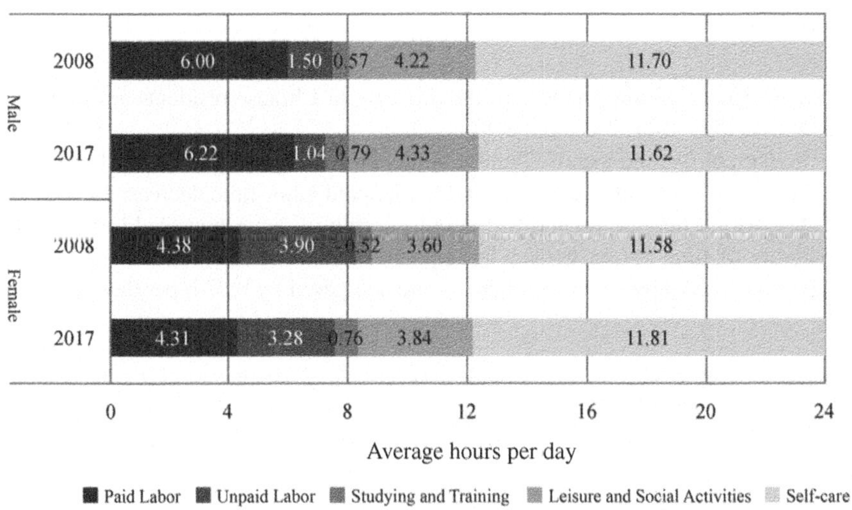

Fig. 2.12 Comparison of average participation length of various activities by gender between 2008 and 2017

and training time increased by 0.23 h per day. Leisure and social time increased by 0.18 h per day; this is related to the residents' higher income and higher pursuit of quality of life. In addition, self-care time increased slightly.

From 2008 to 2017, there were both similarities and differences in the changes in the time use patterns of Chinese men and women, with a general trend of narrowing gender differences. The paid labor time increased for men but decreased for women

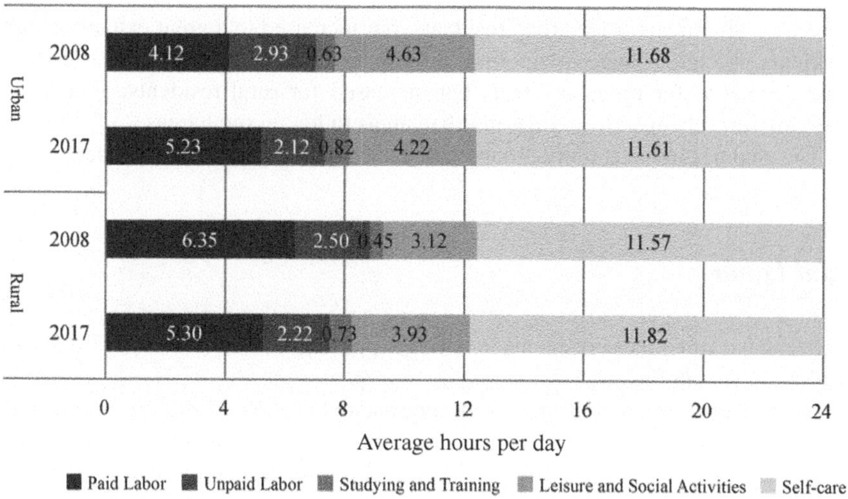

Fig. 2.13 Comparison of average participation length of various activities by urban and rural areas between 2008 and 2017

with a greater gap in gender differences. The unpaid labor time decreased significantly for both men and women; the decrease was greater for women, and the gender gap narrowed. The division of work within the household has returned to the traditional direction of "men's work centers around outside, while women's work centers on home". Total work (paid + unpaid) time decreased for both men and women, but the decrease for men (0.24 h) was much smaller than that for women (0.69 h), resulting in a significant decrease in the gender difference in total work hours. Studying and training time for both men and women increased significantly, and the gender difference decreased. Leisure and social time increased for both men and women; the increase was greater for women, with narrowing gender differences. Self-care time decreased for men and increased for women; as a result, self-care time changed from the situation where men spent more time on self-care than women to women spending more time than men.

It can be found that the pattern of time use in urban and rural China has had different changes from 2008 to 2017, with the general trend of a significant reduction in urban–rural differences. The paid labor time increased significantly for urban residents, but decreased significantly for rural residents; the initial huge urban–rural differences almost disappeared; this reflects the heavier urban workload and that the increased agricultural mechanization reduced work time input in agriculture. Unpaid labor time decreased significantly for both urban and rural residents; however, the decrease was greater for urban residents, making the unpaid labor time change from a high level in urban areas to a low level in rural areas. The difference between urban and rural areas in total work (paid labor + unpaid labor) time decreased significantly. The studying and training time for both urban and rural residents increased significantly, and the difference between urban and rural areas decreased. Leisure and social time decreased significantly for urban residents, but increased to a great extent for rural residents; the initial huge urban–rural difference decreased significantly. Self-care time decreased for urban residents but increased for rural residents; as a result, self-care time changed from high in urban areas to low in rural areas.

The changes in the activity groups under each division are described below.

Paid Labor

The time use of Chinese residents in terms of paid labor in 2008 and 2017 is shown in Table 2.18 and Fig. 2.14.

It can be observed that the paid labor time had only increased slightly and changed little from 2008 to 2017, but there are contrasting changes in the patterns of time use of the various types of paid labor. Job hours rose significantly by 1.08 h per day. The reasons for this are that (1) job hours were rising in both urban and rural areas; (2) job hours were much higher in urban areas than in rural areas, and the rapid increase in the level of urbanization (from 47.0 to 58.5%) had led to an increase in the weight of urban areas. Household production and management time dropped sharply by 1.00 h per day, and the time for the household primary, secondary and tertiary industries all dropped sharply. The reasons for this may be (1) mechanization saves agricultural labor time; (2) the 2008 survey was conducted in May of that year, which was the busy farming season; while the 2017 survey was conducted in July and August, with a decrease in the level of agricultural activities; and (3) the household production and management time in the rural areas was much higher than that in the urban areas, while the rapid urbanization made the weighing of rural areas decrease.

Table 2.18 Comparison of average participation length of paid labor between 2008 and 2017. Unit: hours/day

Year	Activity	Total	Male	Female	Urban	Rural
2008	Paid labor	5.18	6.00	4.38	4.12	6.35
	Job	2.95	3.55	2.37	3.92	1.87
	Household production and management	2.23	2.45	2.02	0.20	4.48
	#Household primary industry	1.82	1.92	1.73	0.02	3.83
	#Household secondary industry	0.17	0.22	0.10	0.02	0.32
	#Household tertiary industry	0.25	0.32	0.18	0.17	0.33
2017	Paid labor	5.26	6.22	4.31	5.23	5.30
	Job	4.03	4.84	3.23	4.84	3.14
	Household production and management	1.23	1.39	1.08	0.39	2.16
	#Household primary industry	1.07	1.21	0.93	0.24	1.99
	#Household secondary industry	0.02	0.03	0.02	0.02	0.02
	#Household tertiary industry	0.14	0.15	0.13	0.13	0.15

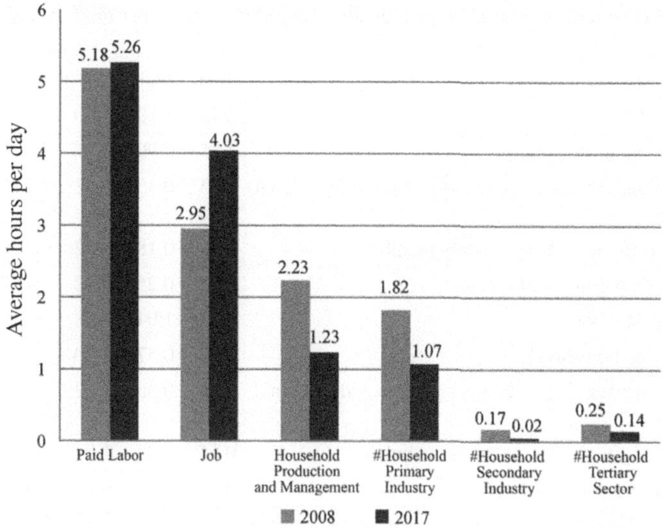

Fig. 2.14 Comparison of average participation length of various types of paid labor between 2008 and 2017

From 2008 to 2017, both men's and women's job hours had risen significantly, while household production and management time fell significantly. The proportion of household primary industry time to the total paid labor time decreased from 0.32 to 0.19 for men and from 0.39 to 0.22 for women. Considering that agricultural (primary industry) labor is less well-paid than non-agricultural work, the quality of paid labor improved significantly for both men and women, and more so for women.

In 2008, rural residents' agricultural labor hours were one time higher than wage labor (job) hours, while in 2017 the relation was reversed, with wage labor hours taking over one hour higher than agricultural labor hours. It is evident that the quality of paid labor of rural residents has improved significantly.

Unpaid Labor

In 2008 and 2017, the time use of Chinese residents in terms of unpaid labor is shown in Table 2.19 and Fig. 2.15.

It can be found that there had been a significant decrease in the time spent on unpaid labor from 2008 to 2017, but there were different patterns of time use for each type of unpaid labor. The time spent doing housework decreased by 0.56 h per day. This reflects the development of market services, the outsourcing of some household chores, and the popularity of time-saving household appliances. Time spent caring for underage family members rose by 0.30 h per day, an increase of nearly a factor of one. Possible reasons for this are (1) greater emphasis on child

Table 2.19 Comparison of average participation length of unpaid labor in 2008 and 2017. Unit: hours/day

Year	Activity	Total	Male	Female	Urban	Rural
2008	Unpaid labor	2.72	1.50	3.90	2.93	2.50
	#Doing housework	1.85	0.90	2.77	1.88	1.83
	#Caring for family members and provide external help	0.53	0.35	0.72	0.58	0.50
	#Caring for underage family members	0.35	0.18	0.52	0.33	0.37
	#Buying goods and services	0.33	0.25	0.42	0.47	0.17
2017	Unpaid labor	2.17	1.04	3.28	2.12	2.22
	#Doing housework	1.29	0.57	2.00	1.20	1.39
	#Caring for family members and provide external help	0.74	0.36	1.12	0.76	0.72
	#Caring for underage family members	0.65	0.28	1.03	0.65	0.65
	#Buying goods and services	0.14	0.11	0.17	0.16	0.11

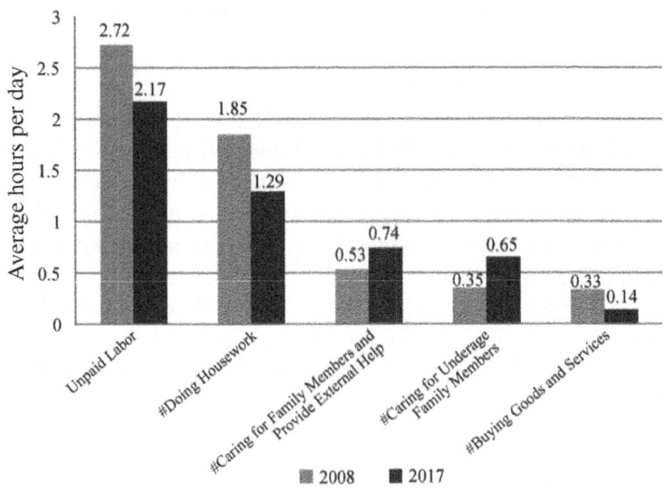

Fig. 2.15 Comparison of average participation length of various types of unpaid labor in 2008 and 2017

caring as living standards improve, and (2) an increase in the number of children in the family due to the opening of the second-child policy. Shopping time decreased by 0.19 h per day, a decrease of more than 50%, which may be related to the rise of online shopping.

From 2008 to 2017, the pattern of change in unpaid labor time by sub-item has been identical for men and women, and urban and rural residents.

Studying and Training

In 2008 and 2017, the time use of Chinese residents in terms of studying and training is shown in Table 2.20 and Fig. 2.16.

It can be observed that there had been a significant rise in the time spent on studying and training from 2008 to 2017, with the same change in the pattern of time use for both types of getting educated and training. The time spent in education rose by 0.20 h per day. Possible reasons for this are (1) the increase in high school, college, and graduate school enrollment, and (2) the competitive pressures for higher education that led students to increase their study time. Training time rose by a factor of one, although the absolute time remained low.

Table 2.20 Comparison of the average participation length of studying and training between 2008 and 2017. Unit: hours/day

Year	Activity	Total	Male	Female	Urban	Rural
2008	Studying and training	0.55	0.57	0.52	0.63	0.45
	#Get educated	0.53	0.55	0.48	0.58	0.45
	#Train	0.02	0.02	0.03	0.05	0
2017	Studying and training	0.78	0.79	0.76	0.82	0.73
	#Get educated	0.73	0.75	0.72	0.77	0.70
	#Train	0.04	0.04	0.04	0.05	0.03

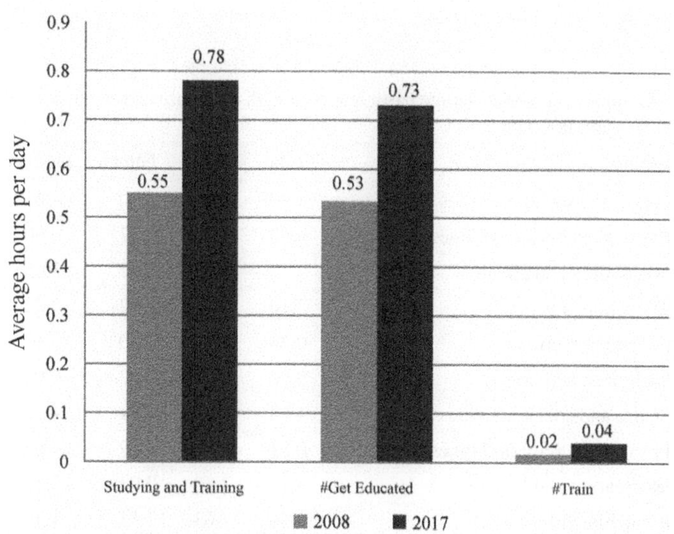

Fig. 2.16 Comparison of the average participation length of various types of studying and training between 2008 and 2017

From 2008 to 2017, the participation length of education and training increased for both men and women, and for both urban and rural residents. Among them, the increase was greater for women and rural residents, resulting in a significant decrease in both the gender and urban–rural differences in time spent on education and training.

Leisure and Social Activities

In 2008 and 2017, the time use of Chinese residents in terms of leisure and social activities is shown in Table 2.21 and Fig. 2.17.

It can be found that the time for leisure and social activities of residents had increased significantly from 2008 to 2017. Overall, high-quality leisure and social time had increased and low-quality leisure and social time had decreased. Exercise and fitness time rose by 0.13 h per day, up by as much as 1/3; this may be related to people pursuing quality of life and caring more about physical health after getting rich. The time spent watching TV dropped by 0.52 h per day, a drop of up to 1/4; the time spent on recreation and leisure other than watching TV rose by 0.51 h per day. After all, there are many recreation and leisure programs now, so naturally, the time spent watching TV will drop. Social interaction time rose slightly.

For both men and women, urban and rural residents, the time spent on exercise and fitness has increased, and the time spent on watching TV decreased. It can be seen that not only people's leisure time has increased, but also the quality of leisure has improved.

Table 2.21 Comparison of the average participation length of leisure and social activities between 2008 and 2017. Unit: hours/day

Year	Activity	Total	Male	Female	Urban	Rural
2008	Leisure and social activities	3.90	4.22	3.60	4.63	3.12
	#Physical exercise and fitness activities	0.38	0.40	0.37	0.60	0.15
	# Recreation and leisure	3.12	3.45	2.82	3.65	2.53
	##Watching TV	2.10	2.18	2.02	2.22	1.95
	#Social interaction	0.38	0.37	0.40	0.37	0.42
	# Religious activities	0.02	0.00	0.02	0.02	0.02
2017	Leisure and social activities	4.08	4.33	3.84	4.22	3.93
	#Physical exercise and fitness activities	0.51	0.55	0.47	0.65	0.36
	# Recreation and leisure	3.11	3.30	2.92	3.15	3.05
	##Watching TV	1.58	1.63	1.53	1.49	1.68
	#Social interaction	0.44	0.46	0.43	0.40	0.50
	# Religious activities	0.02	0.02	0.02	0.02	0.02

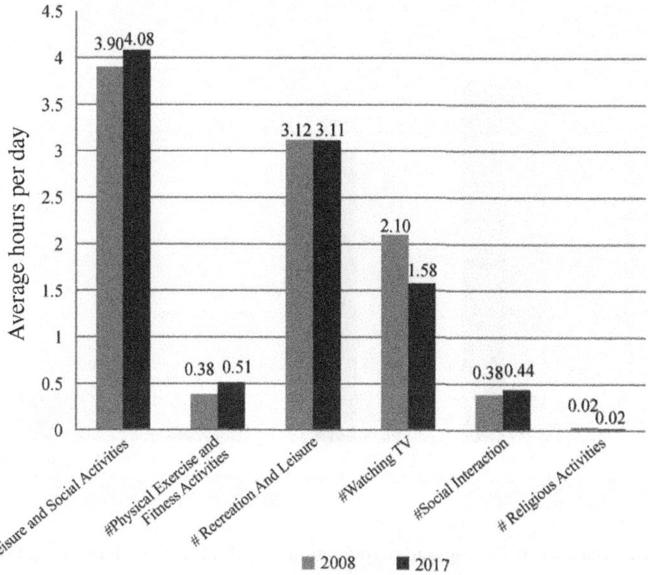

Fig. 2.17 Comparison of the average participation length of various types of leisure and social activities between 2008 and 2017

Self-care

In 2008 and 2017, the time use of Chinese residents in self-care is shown in Table 2.22 and Fig. 2.18.

It can be noticed that people's self-care time has slightly increased from 2008 to 2017. Among them, sleep time rose by 0.44 hours per day, personal hygiene time decreased by 0.25 hours per day, and time spent on dietary activities also decreased slightly.

Table 2.22 Comparison of the average participation length of self-care between 2008 and 2017. Unit: hours/day

Year	Activity	Total	Male	Female	Urban	Rural
2008	Self-care	11.63	11.70	11.58	11.68	11.57
	#Sleep	9.03	9.00	9.07	8.98	9.08
	#Personal hygiene activities	0.77	0.77	0.77	0.83	0.70
	# Dietary activities	1.75	1.83	1.67	1.80	1.70
2017	Self-care	11.71	11.62	11.81	11.61	11.82
	#Sleep	9.47	9.38	9.55	9.36	9.58
	#Personal hygiene activities	0.52	0.50	0.54	0.55	0.49
	# Dietary activities	1.72	1.73	1.72	1.70	1.75

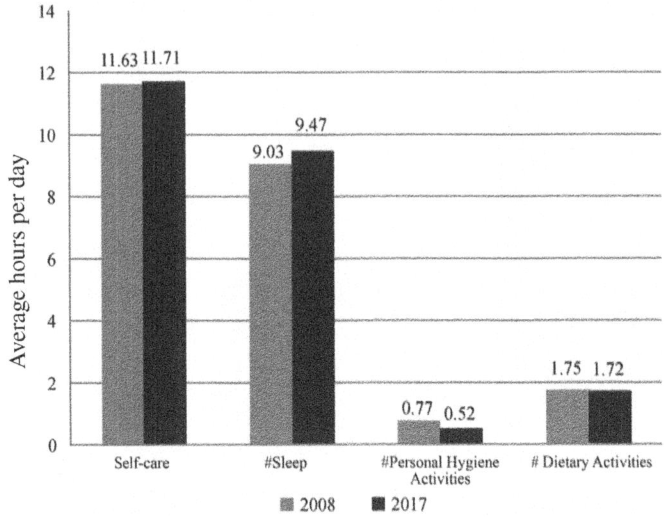

Fig. 2.18 Comparison of the average participation length of various types of self-care between 2008 and 2017

For both men and women, urban and rural residents, sleep time increased and personal hygiene time decreased.

Comparison of Time Use Between China and Other Countries

Because countries are at different stages of development and have different cultural backgrounds, time use can also differ. This section compares the time use differences between China and 10 major developed countries, one transitional country, and three developing countries based on comparable international Time Use Survey data. The sample countries include all developed countries with a population of more than 20 million. The data for these countries are obtained from the Organization for Economic Cooperation and Development (OECD) website.[2] The basic information of the Time Use Survey is shown in Table 2.23.

Since most countries present time use data taken from the samples aged 15–64 years old, this section calculates time use data from the samples aged 15–64 years old of the 2017 Chinese Time Use Survey. A few countries (Australia, Poland, China 2008) present different age groups and their data are less comparable. For comparison purposes, the average values for the 28 countries in OECD are also included in the following analysis.

[2] http://Stats.oecd.org/Index.aspx?datasetcode=TIME_USE.

Table 2.23 Basic information on TUS across countries

Country type	Country name	Year of the survey	Age group
Developed countries	The United States of America	2016	15–64
	Canada	2015	15–64
	Australia[a]	2006	15+
	Germany	2012/2013	15–64
	France	2009/2010	15–64
	The United Kingdom	2014/2015	15–64
	Italy	2013/2014	15–64
	Spain	2009/2010	15–64
	Japan	2016	15–64
	Republic of Korea	2009	15–64
Transitional country	Poland[a]	2013	15 +
Developing countries	China 2008[a]	2008	15–64
	China 2017	2017	15–64
	India	1998/1999	15–64
	Mexico	2014	15–64
	South Africa	2010	15–64

Note [a] The data presented in this section for China in 2008 differ slightly from the data in Section two of this chapter due to different data sources and aggregation methods

Paid Labor

The average participation length of paid labor and the gender differences between countries are shown in Figs. 2.19, 2.20, and 2.21.

It can be observed that Chinese residents have the longest paid labor time among the countries in the sample, more than one time higher than Italy, which ranks last. The countries closest to China are Japan and the Republic of Korea, two developed East Asian countries, and Mexico and India, two developing countries. In terms of hours of paid labor by gender, Chinese men are second only to Mexico and Japan, and Chinese women rank at the top. In terms of gender differences in hours of paid labor, all countries in the sample are higher for men than women. China ranks at the top, just below Mexico, India, Japan, Korea, and Australia.

Unpaid Labor

The average participation length of unpaid labor of residents and the gender differences among countries are shown in Figs. 2.22, 2.23, and 2.24.

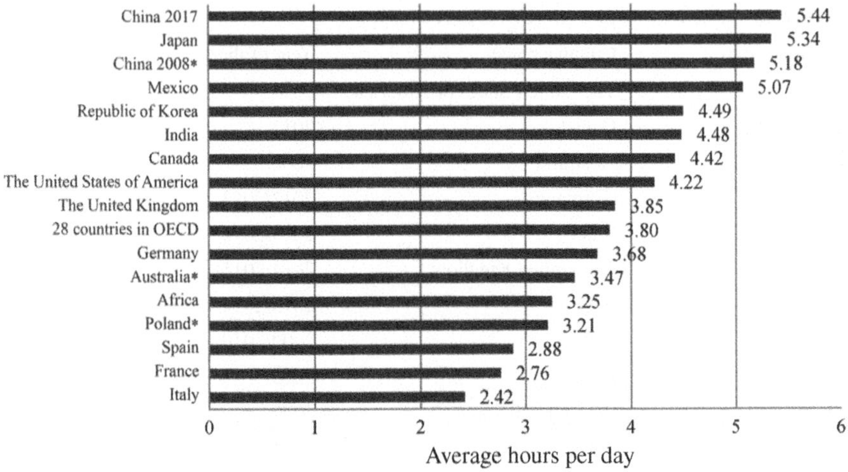

Fig. 2.19 Comparison of average participation length of paid labor across countries

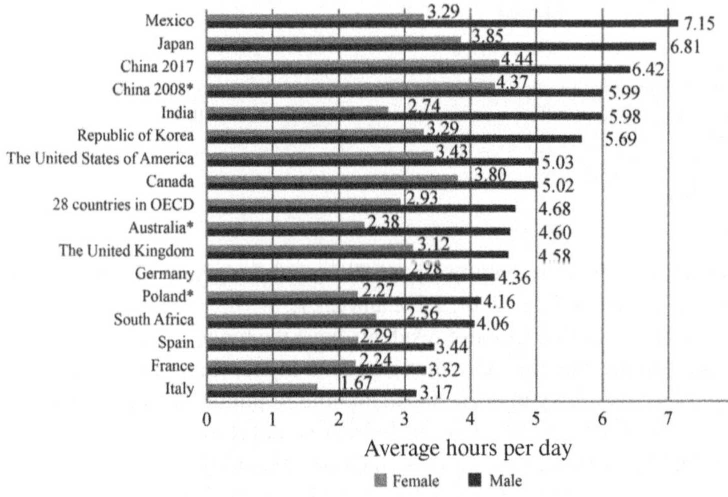

Fig. 2.20 Average participation length of paid labor by gender across countries

It can be found that, among the sample countries, Chinese residents have the shortest duration of unpaid labor, which is less than half of that of the highest-ranked Mexico. The closest to China are Japan and the Republic of Korea. In terms of unpaid labor time by gender, Chinese men are only higher than Japan, Korea, and India, and Chinese women are the lowest. In terms of gender differences in unpaid labor hours, all countries in the sample are higher for females than males. China ranks in the middle, much lower than India and Mexico, and significantly lower than Japan, South Korea, and Italy.

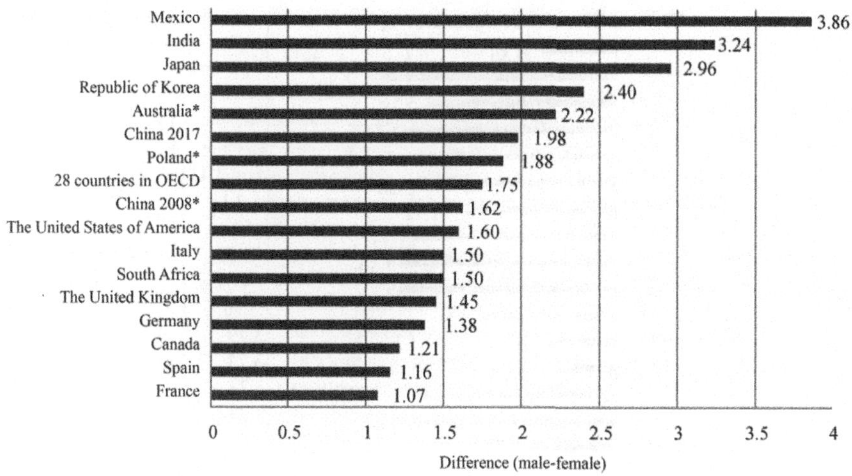

Fig. 2.21 Gender differences in average participation length of paid labor across countries

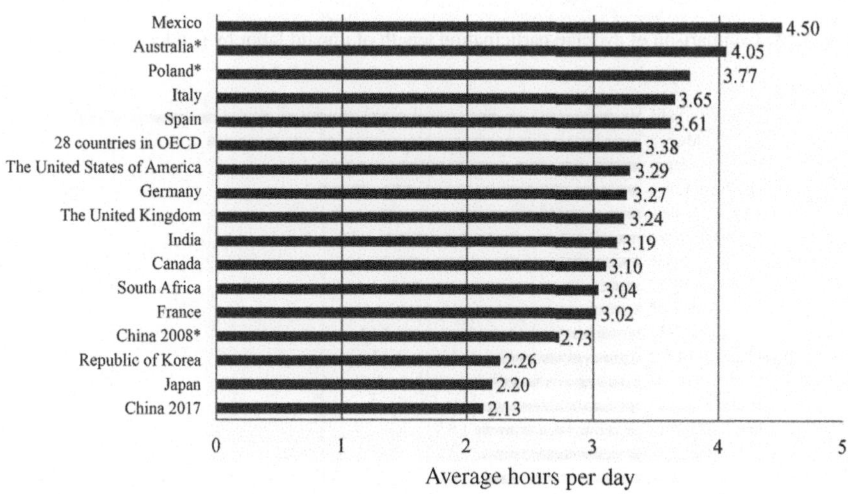

Fig. 2.22 Comparison of average participation length of unpaid labor across countries

Studying and Training

The average participation length of studying and training of residents and their gender differences by country are shown in Figs. 2.25, 2.26, and 2.27.

It can be found that, among the sample countries, Chinese residents rank third in terms of learning and training time, only lower than the Republic of Korea and Mexico. In terms of studying and training time by gender, Chinese men and women both rank third, just below the Republic of Korea and Mexico. In terms of gender

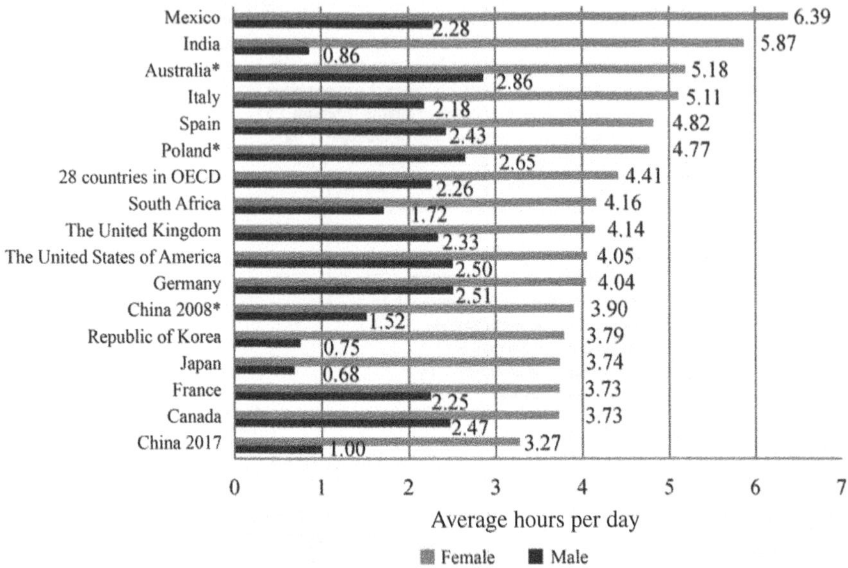

Fig. 2.23 Comparison of average participation length of unpaid labor by gender across countries

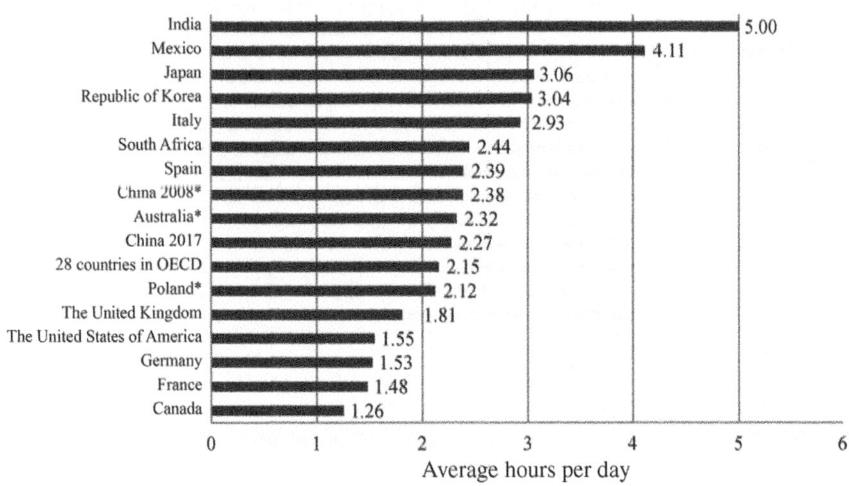

Fig. 2.24 Gender differences in average participation length of unpaid labor across countries

differences in studying and training time, men are higher than women in most sample countries. China ranks fourth, significantly lower than India and South Africa, slightly lower than the UK, and higher than most developed countries.

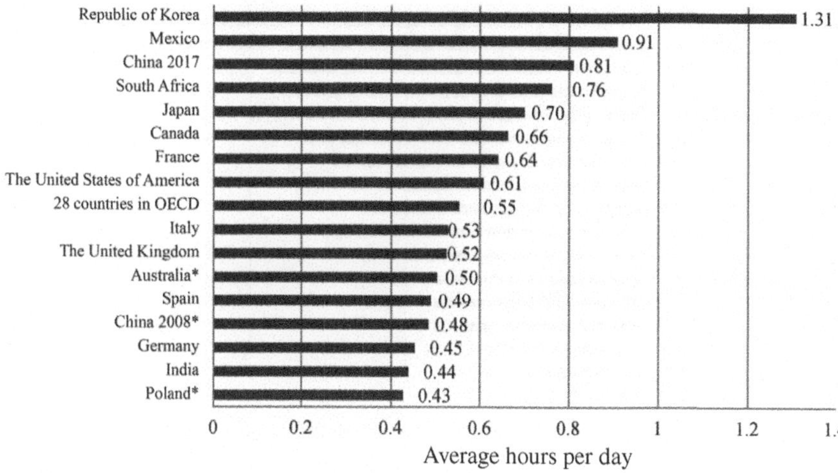

Fig. 2.25 Comparison of the average participation length of studying and training across countries

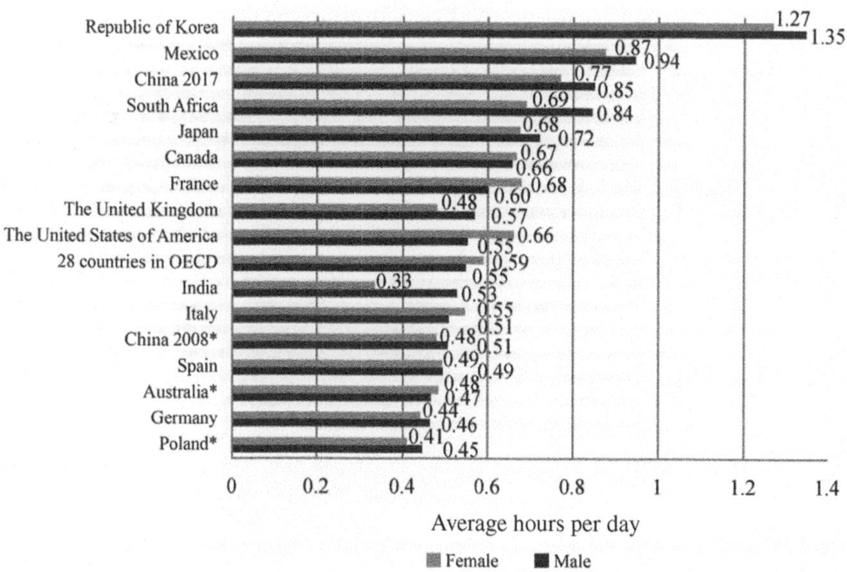

Fig. 2.26 The average participation length of studying and training by gender across countries

Leisure and Social Activities

The average participation length of leisure and social activities and the gender differences across countries are shown in Figs. 2.28, 2.29, and 2.30.

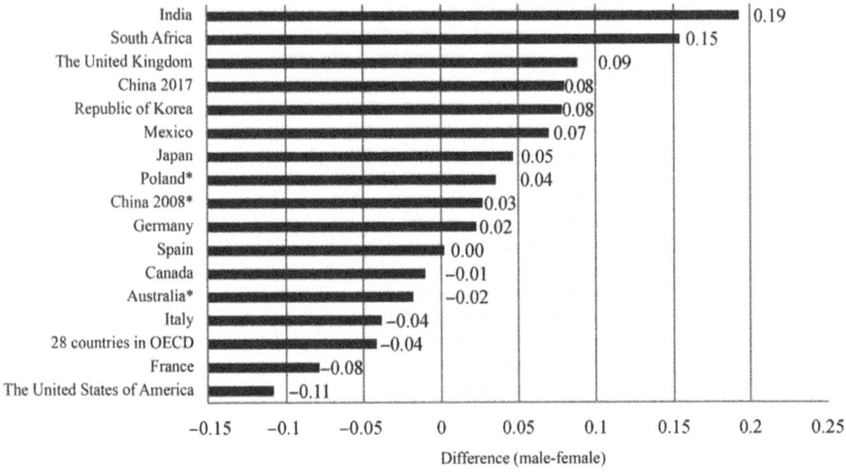

Fig. 2.27 Gender differences in the average participation length of studying and training across countries

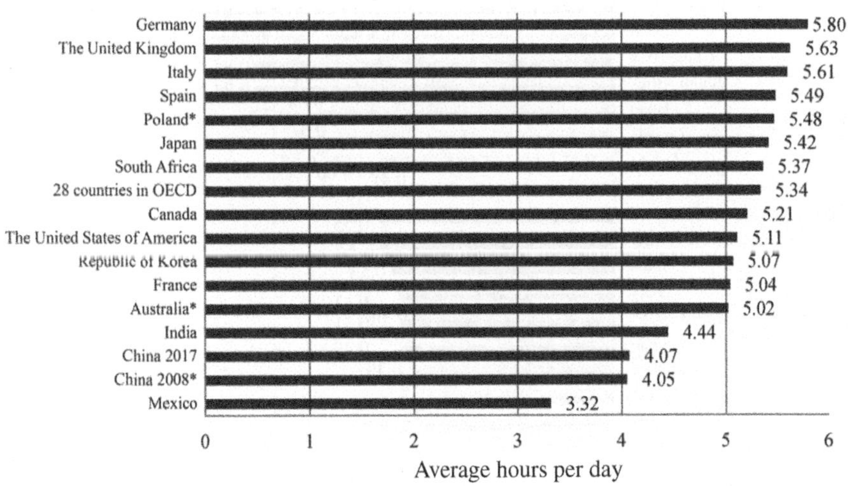

Fig. 2.28 Comparison of the average participation length of leisure and social activities across countries

It can be found that among the sample countries, Chinese residents rank the second lowest in terms of leisure social time, just above Mexico. In terms of the time spent on leisure and social activities by gender, both Chinese males and females rank second to last, only higher than Mexico. In terms of gender differences in the time spent on leisure and social activities, males are higher than females in all countries in the sample. China ranks fourth from the bottom, just above Japan, Australia, and Mexico.

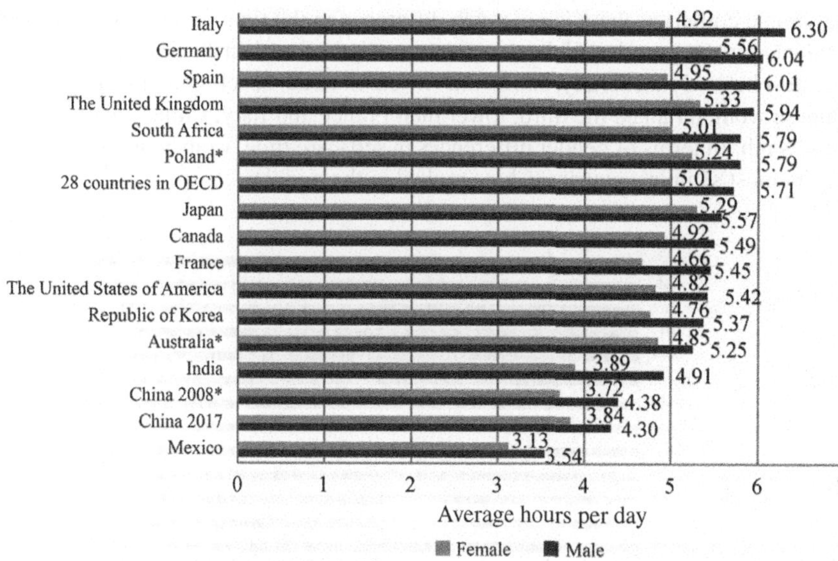

Fig. 2.29 The average participation length of leisure and social activities by gender across countries

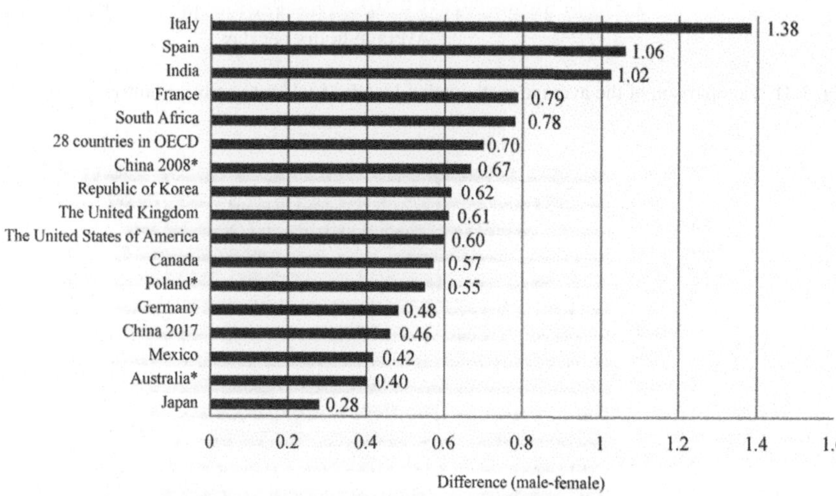

Fig. 2.30 Gender differences in the average participation length of leisure and social activities across countries

Self-care

The average participation length of self-care for residents and their gender differences across countries are shown in Figs. 2.31, 2.32, and 2.33. It can be found that among the sample countries, there is not much difference in the time spent on self-care for residents across countries. Chinese residents rank the fourth in the time spent on self-care, just below France, Italy, and South Africa. In terms of self-care time by gender, Chinese women ranked the third, lower than France and Italy; Chinese men ranked the seventh. In terms of gender differences in self-care time, women are higher than men in most sample countries. China ranked in the middle.

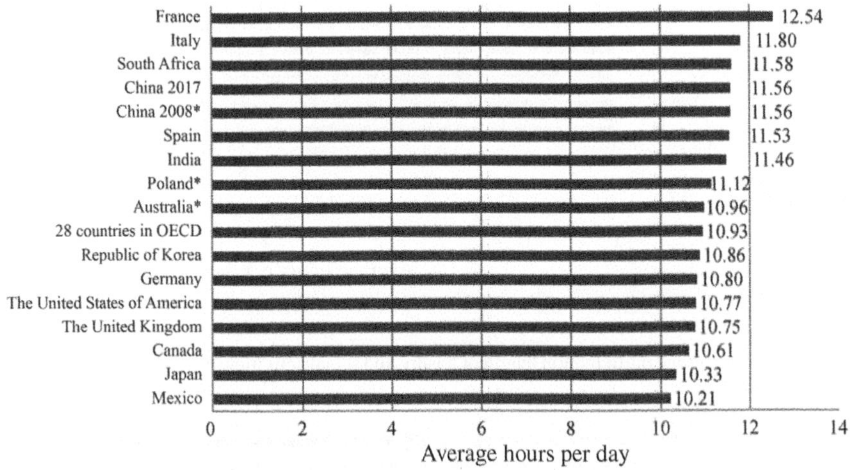

Fig. 2.31 Comparison of the average participation length of self-care across countries

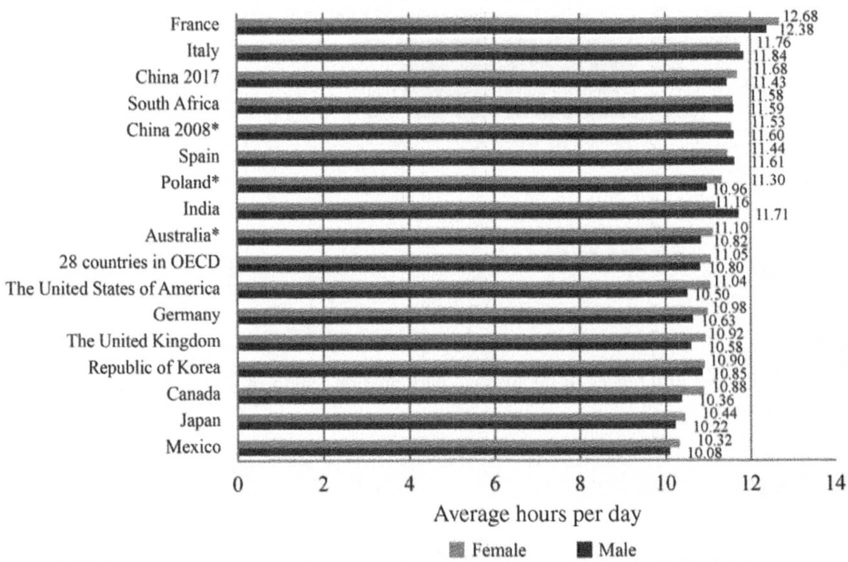

Fig. 2.32 The average participation length of self-care by gender across countries

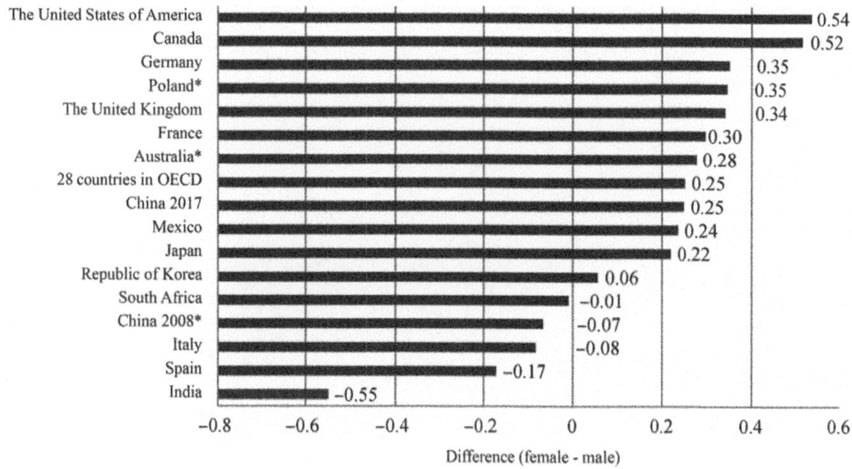

Fig. 2.33 Gender differences in the average participation length of self-care across acountries

Summary

This chapter presents China's time use in 2017 and compares it with China's situation in 2008 and with other countries. The following conclusions are drawn.

First, in total labor, Chinese men are more engaged in paid labor, while women are more engaged in unpaid labor. The total labor time of women is slightly higher than that of men. The average length of leisure socialization decreases and then increases with age, and tends to decrease with education level.

Second, compared with 2008, the time spent on paid labor in China changed little in 2017, and the time spent on unpaid labor decreased by 0.54 h per day. But the time spent caring for underage family members increased significantly. The time spent on leisure and social activities increased by 0.44 h per day, and the structure of these activities was optimized. The gender difference in time use is narrowing, and the difference between urban and rural areas was significantly reduced. This reflects the rising living standard of residents and their greater pursuit of quality of life, as well as the increasing urbanization rate and the change in industrial structure.

Third, compared with 14 other countries, Chinese residents rank first in hours of paid labor, while they rank last in hours of unpaid labor. Chinese residents rank first in the time spent on studying and training and self-care, and second in the time spent on leisure and social activities.

Part II
The Busy Chinese: Balancing Work and Family

Chapter 3
Overtime Workers

Employment is the main way for most people in modern society to obtain income and social recognition. Providing good working conditions for the employed[1] is one of the important elements of the Decent Work Agenda by the International Labor Organization (ILO). In the time dimension, Decent Work Time is one of the indicators of Decent Work and a manifestation of good working conditions.[2]

In China, overtime work is common among workers, whether they are employees of enterprises, commonly known as "wage earners", or employees of government departments, institutions, and enterprises, commonly known as "(people with) iron rice bowls". Overtime work, namely extra and extended work, means that employees' work time exceeds the standard work time stipulated by law. According to the Labor Law of the People's Republic of China (hereinafter referred to as Labor Law), a system for work time has been implemented, in which the net daily work time does not exceed 8 h and the average weekly work time does not exceed 44 h. According to the Labor Law, a worker's net daily work time[3] once exceeds 8 h is defined as overtime work. This chapter focuses on the overtime work of Chinese wage earners[4] from the dimension of overtime work rate.[5]

The data used in this chapter are from the 2017 Chinese Time Use Survey. The sample for the study included all wage earners whose employment status was an employee (excluding employers, self-employed, and household helpers) and those who were 16 years old and above. It totaled 7,178 people, of whom 4,072 were men and 3,106 were women. There were 5,894 urban residents and 1,284 rural residents.

[1] Refers to employed work in the labor market (excluding self-employment).

[2] Liangshu Qi, Xinli An, Xiaoyuan Dong, "Paid Work of China's Residents from the Time-use Statistics", *Statistical Research*, 2012 (4).

[3] Net daily work time refers to the work time excluding transportation, work breaks and related waiting activities, on-the-job training, job hunting, and resignation.

[4] Wage earners are workers in the labor market who receive wage income by being employed. In other words, the employment status is an employee (non-employer).

[5] The overtime work rate is the ratio of the number of people with net work time greater than 8 h to the number of people working.

F. Du et al., *Chinese People's Time Use and Their Quality of Life*,
https://doi.org/10.1007/978-981-99-5526-8_3

According to China's working age population, the legal working age for males is from 16 to 60 years old and from 16 to 55 years old for females. In the data used in this chapter, male employees aged 16–60 years old accounted for 92.0% of the total male employees, and female employees aged 16–55 years old accounted for 91.9% of the total female employees.

Overview of the Overtime Work

Generally speaking, from the start of work to the end of work, the average total daily work[6] time of Chinese wage earners was 7.7 h; after deducting the time spent on activities such as transportation, drinking, smoking, resting, and going to the toilet, the average net daily work time was 7.0 h. Compared with the data in 2008, the average total daily work time increased by 1.8 h, and the average net daily work time increased by 2.3 h. The net weekly work time of Chinese wage earners was 48.9 h.[7] Compared with OECD countries (see Fig. 3.1), the average net weekly work time of Chinese workers was higher than that of most developed countries, such as the United States, the United Kingdom, and Germany, and comparable to some developing countries, such as Colombia, Mexico, and Turkey.

In terms of gender, men's average total daily work time and average net daily work time were about 38 and 32 min more than women's, respectively. Overall, about 42% of employees worked more than 8 h a day, and the overtime work rate of men was about 45%, which was 6% points higher than that of women. In 2008, the overtime work rate was only 12%, which has increased by 30% points in 9 years. This reflects that Chinese residents have become more stressed at work, busier in life, and that overtime work has become more common.

According to the Labor Law, if it is necessary to extend the work time for special reasons, the extended work time should not exceed 3 h per day under the condition of safeguarding the health of workers. However, as shown in Table 3.1, about 11% of the people worked more than 11 net hours per day on average, and men were higher than women by about 4% points in average daily work time. This indicates that a considerable number of employers ignored the Labor Law provisions and extended the work time beyond 3 h. In addition, about 14% of employees worked before 7 a.m. or after 8 p.m. during non-regular work time. This is another reflection of the seriousness of the overtime work among Chinese "salary men".

[6] *Work* refers to *work and work-related activities* in the activity division of the 2017 China Time-use Survey.

[7] The average net daily work time is multiplied by 7 to calculate the weekly work time.

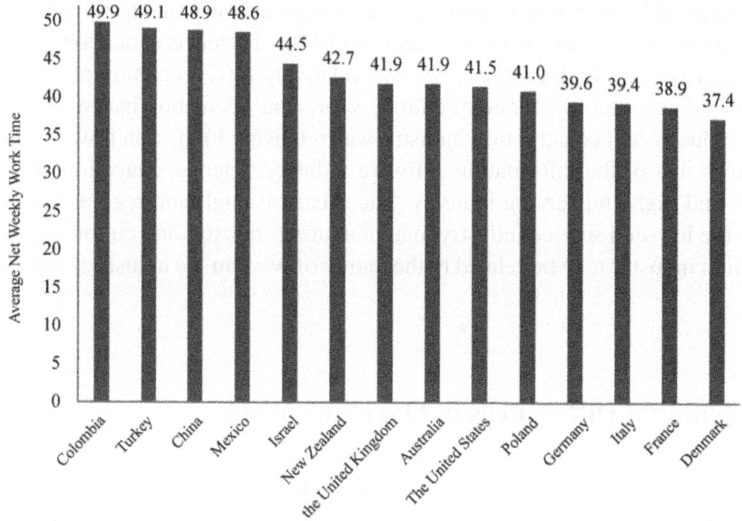

Fig. 3.1 Average net weekly work time in China and OECD Countries (2017). *Source* Data on China is from the 2017 Chinese Time Use Survey (CTUS), and the data on other countries is from https://stats.oecd.org/Index.aspx

Table 3.1 Overtime work by gender

	Countrywide	Male	Female
Number of people working	7178	4072	3106
Average total daily work time (hours)	7.71	7.97	7.34
Average net daily work time[a] (hours)	6.99	7.21	6.68
Overtime work rate[b] (%)	42.2	44.7	38.7
Serious overtime work rate[c] (%)	10.6	12.3	8.2
Non-regular time work rate[d] (%)	14.3	14.6	13.8

Note [a] Refers to the work time excluding transportation, work breaks and related waiting activities, on-the-job training, job hunting, and resignation; [b] Refers to the ratio of the number of people working more than 8 h net to the number of people working; [c] Refers to the ratio of the number of people working more than 11 h to the number of people working; [d] Refers to the ratio of the number of people working during non-regular work time to the number of people working, and non-regular work time refers to the working time before 7 a.m. or after 8 p.m.

Industrial Differences in Overtime Work

As shown in Table 3.2, when analyzed by industry, the average total daily work time of workers in the manufacturing, information and software, and culture, sports and recreation industries is higher than 8 h. The average net daily work time of manufacturing workers was the longest, followed by the culture, sports and recreation industry. The overtime work rate of manufacturing workers was the highest, at about

59%; followed by the cultural, sports and recreation industry, and lastly the construction industry. In comparison, the overtime work rate of science, education, health and social services and high-end services was relatively low, remaining at about 30%. The serious overtime work rate of culture, sports and recreation industry, manufacturing industry and construction industry was relatively high, which was more than two times that of the information software industry, science, education and health society and high-end service industry. The relatively high non-regular hours work rate in the low-end service industry, manufacturing industry and culture, sports and recreation industry may be related to the nature of work in the industries they belong to.

Occupational Differences in Overtime Work

As shown in Table 3.3, in terms of occupation, the average net daily work time of manufacturing workers is the longest, followed by service providers, and then professional and technical staff. The average net daily work time of manufacturing workers was nearly one hour longer than that of clerical staff in state organs, enterprises and institutions. The overtime work rate of manufacturing workers was the highest at 58%, followed by service providers at about 45%. The overtime work rate of manufacturing workers was 1.5 times higher than that of clerical staff in state organs, enterprises and institutions. Manufacturing workers had the highest rate of serious overtime work, followed by service providers. The serious overtime work rate of manufacturing workers was 1.8 times higher than that of the clerical staff of state organs, enterprises and institutions. The non-regular hours work rate of manufacturing workers and service providers is comparable.

Summary

This chapter analyzes the overtime work situation of Chinese wage earners in the dimension of overtime work rate, and draws the following main conclusions and policy recommendations.

First, on the whole, overtime work is common among workers in all industries in China to varying degrees. Overloaded tasks, performance appraisal pressure, economic pressure, career promotion pressure, and overtime culture are the main reasons for overtime work of workers.[8] No matter what the cause is, if workers work too long, they are bound to squeeze out the time to meet their basic needs such as rest, recreation and leisure, which means they will fall into the dilemma of

[8] Xuduo Meng, Xin Wang, "Causes of Overtime Work and Characteristics of Work Time for Corporate Employees", *Research on Economics and Management*, 2015 (12).

Table 3.2 Overtime work by industries

	Manufacturing	Construction industry	Low-end service industry[a]	High-end service industry[b]	Information software industry[c]	Culture, sports and recreation[d]	Science, education, health and social[c]
Number of people working	1095	659	1196	441	176	118	1548
Average total daily work time (hours)	8.45	7.83	7.67	7.61	8.13	8.37	6.78
Average net daily work time (hours)	7.75	6.99	7.09	6.69	7.11	7.62	6.11
Overtime work rate (%)	58.8	53.6	40.9	31.9	42.0	54.1	28.3
Serious overtime work rate (%)	13.9	12.1	12.1	5.5	6.6	15.8	5.9
Non-regular time work rate (%)	18.6	4.7	20.8	6.6	13.4	17.5	10.1

Note [a] Refers to the accommodation and catering industry, residential services, repair and other services; [b] Refers to the financial sector, real estate, and rental and business services; [c] Refers to information transmission, software and information technology services and scientific research; [d] Refers to culture, sports and recreation; [e] Refers to scientific research, technical services, education, health, public administration, social security and social organizations

Table 3.3 Overtime work by occupation

	Principal[a]	Clerical staff[b]	Professional and technical staff	Service provider[c]	Manufacturing worker[d]
Number of people working	270	1879	1532	1547	1061
Average total daily work time (hours)	7.28	7.28	7.76	8.00	8.11
Average net daily work time (hours)	6.38	6.59	6.98	7.31	7.51
Overtime work rate (%)	25.6	38.4	35.6	45.4	57.8
Serious overtime work rate (%)	3.5	8.5	7.2	13.5	15.2
Non-regular time work rate (%)	3.4	11.8	11.9	18.5	18.2

Note [a] Refers to the heads of Party organs, state organs, mass and social organizations, enterprises and public institutions; [b] Refers to clerical and related personnel of the Party organs, state organs, groups and social organizations, enterprises and institutions; [c] Refers to service providers of social production and living services; [d] Refers to manufacturing and related personnel

the so-called "Time-poor".[9] In the long run, excessive overtime work will damage workers' physical and mental health, and may even lead to "death from overwork". Therefore, this phenomenon of normal overtime work needs to arouse the government and society's high attention, and a restrictive, reasonable and scientific work time system should be established through legislation and other institutional arrangements to regulate certain reasonable overtime work and curb illegal and unreasonable overtime work.[10]

Second, overtime work is more serious for workers of informal sectors than those of formal sectors, although the Labor Law stipulates that the net work time of workers should not exceed 8 h per day and 44 h per week. If employers need to extend the working hours of employees, they should pay wages higher than the employees' normal work time according to the corresponding standards. However, some companies or employers often force workers to work overtime on the grounds of catching up with the work schedule, etc., and then reduce the working hours after the schedule is done so that the average work time does not exceed 8 h, as stipulated by the Labor Law, so as to circumvent the payment of overtime wages to workers. Since workers in informal sectors do not have formal labor contracts with the employer, their legal

[9] Vickery, Clair, "The Time-poor: A New Look at Poverty". *Journal of Human Resources*, 1977, 12 (1).

[10] Zhengmo Guo, "Can Overtime Work in Enterprises with Chinese Characteristics Be Considered as 'Decent Work'—Overtime Work and the Behavior Analysis of Both Parties of the Internal Labor Market", *Social Science Research*, 2015 (4).

rights and interests are even more difficult to be protected. The 2017 China Household Finance Survey (CHFS) data show that about 56% of overtime workers in China did not receive the overtime wages stipulated by the Labor Law. Therefore, in order to effectively protect workers' rights and interests, efforts should be made to strengthen the performance and supervision of the Labor Law, the Law of the People's Republic of China on Employment Contracts and other laws and regulations, with a special focus on the informal sectors.

Chapter 4
Gender Differences in Unpaid Labor

"Unpaid labor refers to service activities performed by individuals at home or in the community to satisfy final consumption without direct monetary return, mainly including housework, care for the elderly, children and the sick, and voluntary activities".[1] As a productive input to human resources, unpaid labor is not only essential to improving the health and well-being of the population, but also determines the quality and quantity of a country's present and future labor supply, thereby influencing the speed and sustainability of economic growth. Thus, unpaid labor is by nature as important to national welfare as market-based economic activities.[2] Neglecting unpaid labor leads to insufficient investment in household consumption and care for children and the elderly, which affects people's living standards and health welfare, and is thus detrimental to social and economic development.[3]

In most countries around the world, unpaid labor is predominantly performed by women. The responsibility of women's unpaid labor affects their employment opportunities, career choices, promotion prospects and wages, placing them in a disadvantageous position in the labor market. A large body of literature shows that unpaid labor has a negative effect on labor earnings for both men and women. This effect is known as the *penalty effects of housework*. Moreover, the negative effect of unpaid labor on married men's income is much less than that of married women. This is because the effect of unpaid labor on income has a threshold effect,[4] and different types of unpaid labor have different effects on income. Besides, men's unpaid labor is shorter and has more flexible time arrangements. Numerous empirical studies from the United States, Canada, Germany, and other countries have also found that

[1] Xinli An, Xiaoyuan, "Measurement of the Total Value of Unpaid Labor in China and Its Policy Implications", *Chinese Women's Movement*, 2012 (7).

[2] Ibid.

[3] Zhaoping Wang, Jian Zhang, "A New Estimate of the Value of Unpaid Housework", *Statistics & Decision*, 2015 (5).

[4] The threshold effect here means that unpaid labor has no effect on labor income when the duration of unpaid labor is low.

F. Du et al., *Chinese People's Time Use and Their Quality of Life*,
https://doi.org/10.1007/978-981-99-5526-8_4

the wages of women with children are much lower than those of women without children, which is referred to in the literature as the *motherhood wage penalty*. At the same time, for employed women, the "double burden" of work and family leaves them with insufficient time and energy to devote themselves to learning, training, leisure, and social activities, which not only hinders the accumulation of their human and social capital, but also affects their physical and mental health. In summary, gender differences in the participation length and type of unpaid labor are the main causes of gender inequality, especially in the labor market.[5] The negative impact of unpaid labor on women's own development will further reduce women's willingness to marry and have children, leading to a declining birthrate and a series of social problems such as insufficient labor supply and aging.[6] In view of this, Goal Five of the United Nations 2030 Sustainable Development Goals[7] proposes to achieve gender equality and empower all women and girls by recognizing and valuing unpaid care and domestic work through the provision of public services, infrastructure and social protection policies and the promotion of shared responsibility within the household and the family.

This chapter uses the 2017 Chinese Time Use Survey data to analyze gender differences in unpaid labor in China. Because of the correlation between gender differences and other social differences, the forms of gender differences vary in different social groups. Based on this, this chapter analyzes gender differences in unpaid labor in four aspects: urban and rural division, age, education level, and household income. This chapter answers the following questions: how do Chinese households distribute unpaid labor between men and women? How do gender differences differ across groups? Which social groups have the heaviest burden of unpaid labor and the largest gender differences? The answers to these questions can help improve our understanding of the division of unpaid labor in households and help the government formulate relevant policies in a more targeted manner.

Defining Unpaid Labor

In this chapter, unpaid labor is divided into two categories of activities: housework, caring for family members and providing external assistance. Housework is further divided into three types of activities: regular daily chores, non-regular daily chores and buying goods and services. Caring for family members and providing external assistance can be divided into three types of activities: caring for minors, caring for adults, and volunteer activities. The specific classification is shown in Table 4.1.

[5] Walker J. R., "Earnings, Effort, and Work Flexibility of Self-employed Women and Men: The Case of St. Croix County", *Journal of Labor Research*, 2009, 30 (3).

[6] McDonald, Peter, "Gender Equity, Social Institutions and the Future of Fertility", *Journal of Population Research*, 2000, 17 (1).

[7] On September 15th, 2015, the 193 member states of the United Nations formally adopted 17 Sustainable Development Goals to guide global development efforts for the period from 2015 to 2030.

Table 4.1 Various types of activities of unpaid labor

Division	Activity type	Description
Housework	Regular daily chores	Cooking
		Washing the dishes
		Cleaning
		Laundry, sorting and making clothes
	Non-regular daily chores	Keeping pets
		Small scale DIY renovations, maintenance and repairs
		Arrangements for family affairs
		Other housekeeping activities
	Buying goods and services	Shopping, repairing electrical appliances, haircutting, medical treatment, and conducting business, etc.
Caring for family members and providing external assistance	Caring for minors	Caring for minor family members
		Caring for minor relatives
	Caring for adults	Caring for adult family members
		Caring for adult relatives
	Volunteer activities	Unpaid household help for other families
		Community service and public welfare activities

The survey data used in this chapter are from the 2017 Chinese Time Use Survey, and the study population is Chinese residents aged 16 years and above. The main reasons for excluding the sample under 16 years old are as follows. (1) The average participation length of unpaid labor and the participation rate of residents under 16 years old are at a very low level. (2) From the perspective of cognition, people are accustomed to contrasting unpaid labor with paid labor, and 16-year-old is the lower limit of the national legal employment age, so 16-year-old is taken as the lower limit of the sample age. The study samples in this chapter contain 26,770 people, of which 12,857 are men and 13,913 are women.

Basic Situation of Unpaid Labor

After more than half a century of efforts since the founding of the People's Republic of China, women have made great improvements in education, employment and wages. Their social status is constantly rising, and the gap in men is gradually narrowing.

However, there are still obvious gender differences and inequitable distribution of unpaid labor within a family.[8] In this section, the author analyzes the gender differences in unpaid labor nationwide and compares them with the time use data from the National Bureau of Statistics in 2008.

The Gender Difference of Unpaid Labor Is Huge

As shown from the statistics in Table 4.2, women bear the majority of unpaid labor. Nationally, the average length of unpaid labor per day for women was 3.25 h, compared with 1.10 h for men, and the average participation length of unpaid labor per day for women was 2.95 times that of men. The participation rate of women in unpaid labor was 77.4%, 36.2% points higher than that of men. In addition to volunteering, the average length and participation rate of women in all household chores were higher than those of men, and the average length of women's regular daily chores was 3.77 times that of men's, and the average length of women's care for minors was 3.59 times that of men's. The participation rate of women in regular daily chores was 39.0% points higher than that of men, and the participation rate of women in care for minors was 1.8% points higher than that of men. The average participation length in each household activity showed that the average daily participation length was 4.20 h for women and 2.67 h for men, which was 1.57 times more for women than for men. The average daily participation length of regular daily chores was 2.60 h for women, compared with 1.56 h for men, and this was 1.67 times more for women than men. The average daily participation length of caring for minors was 4.75 h for women, compared with 3.19 h for men, and this was 1.49 times more for women than men. In summary, women were the main bearers of unpaid labor in families, meanwhile, the gender differences in unpaid labor were significant.

Unpaid Labor for Women Is More Inflexible

Not only do men and women differ in the amount of time they spend doing unpaid labor, but also differ in the type of unpaid labor they do. Based on the unpaid labor time binding to the participants, unpaid labor is divided into two categories: low-flexibility unpaid labor including regular daily chores and caring for minors, and flexible unpaid labor including non-regular daily chores, purchase of goods and services, caring for adults, and volunteer activities. As shown in Fig. 4.1, the average participation length of low-flexible unpaid labor was 2.78 h per day for women and 0.75 h per day for men, which was 3.71 times higher for women than for men. The average participation length of regular daily chores was 1.81 h per day for women

[8] Qiyan Wang, Jiajia Wei, "Study on the Differences in Housework Time Between Different Gender Groups", *Journal of Shandong Women's University*, 2018 (1).

Table 4.2 Basic situation of the time use of the unpaid labor of Chinese residents by gender

	Male			Female		
	Average hours per day	Participant duration (hours/day)	Participation rate (%)	Average hours per day	Participant duration (hours/day)	Participation rate (%)
Unpaid labor	1.10	2.67	41.2	3.25	4.20	77.4
#Housework	0.74	2.07	35.7	2.20	3.04	72.4
##Regular daily chores	0.48	1.56	30.7	1.81	2.60	69.7
##Non-regular daily chores	0.13	2.06	6.3	0.20	1.75	11.4
#Purchasing goods and services	0.13	1.24	10.5	0.19	1.71	11.1
#Caring for family members and providing external assistance	0.36	3.40	10.6	1.05	4.69	22.4
##Caring for minors	0.27	3.19	1.9	0.07	3.23	2.2
##Caring for adults	0.06	3.19	1.9	0.07	3.23	2.2
#Volunteer activities	0.03	4.77	0.6	0.02	2.71	0.6

and 0.48 h per day for men, which was 3.77 times higher for women than for men. The average participation length of caring for minors was 0.97 h per day for women and 0.27 h per day for men, which was 3.59 times higher for women than that for men. The average participation length of flexible unpaid labor was 0.48 h per day for women and 0.35 h per day for men, which was 1.37 times more for women than for men. Compared with women, men's participation in unpaid labor was more social, flexible, and less constrained to the liberty of personal time allocation. Studies show that men and women reinforce their respective gender identities through the amount and type of housework each undertakes. After marriage, especially after having children, women are willing to engage in feminine housework, such as cooking, cleaning, taking care of and educating the children, so that they look more like good wives or good mothers.[9] Women's regular daily chores and caring for minors account for a higher proportion of unpaid labor time than men's, which can be a hindrance to women's own development.

[9] Jie Xiao, "Review of the Sociological Research On Housework in China in The Past 20 Years," *Journal of Shandong Women's University*, 2017 (3).

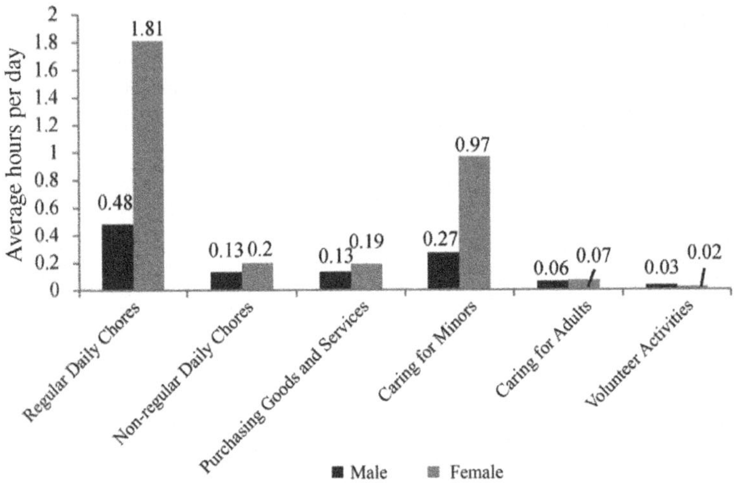

Fig. 4.1 Average participation length of different activity types by gender

The Gender Gap in Unpaid Labor Has Widened Since 2008

By comparing with the data from the 2008 National Bureau of Statistics Time Use Survey, in the nine years from 2008 to 2017, the income level of Chinese residents had increased significantly from the per capita GDP of 24,121 yuan in 2008 to 59,660 yuan in 2017. The value added of the tertiary industry accounted for 51.6% of GDP in 2017, up from 40.1% in 2008.[10] How did rising income levels and changes in industrial structure affect unpaid labor time and gender differences among Chinese residents? Figure 4.2 depicts the changes in the average participation length of the unpaid labor of Chinese residents between 2008 and 2017. The figure shows that compared with the data from 2008, the average participation length of unpaid labor decreased by 0.23 h per day for men, or 17.7%, while that for women decreased by 0.04 h per day, or 1.2%; the average participation length of housework decreased by 0.33 h per day for men, or 32.0%, and decreased by 0.81 h per day for women, or 27.0%. In 2008, compared with men, women spent 2.56 times more time on unpaid labor, 2.91 times more time on housework, and 2.22 times more time caring for family members and providing external assistance. By 2017, these ratios had become 3.07, 3.13 and 2.97 times respectively.

Unpaid labor time and housework time decreased for both men and women, and the decrease rate of men was greater than that of women, while the time spent on family care and external assistance increased, and the increase rate of women was higher than that of men. The difference between men and women in unpaid labor

[10] Source: Statistical Communiqué of the People's Republic of China on the 2008 National Economic and Social Development and Statistical Communiqué of the People's Republic of China on the 2017 National Economic and Social Development.

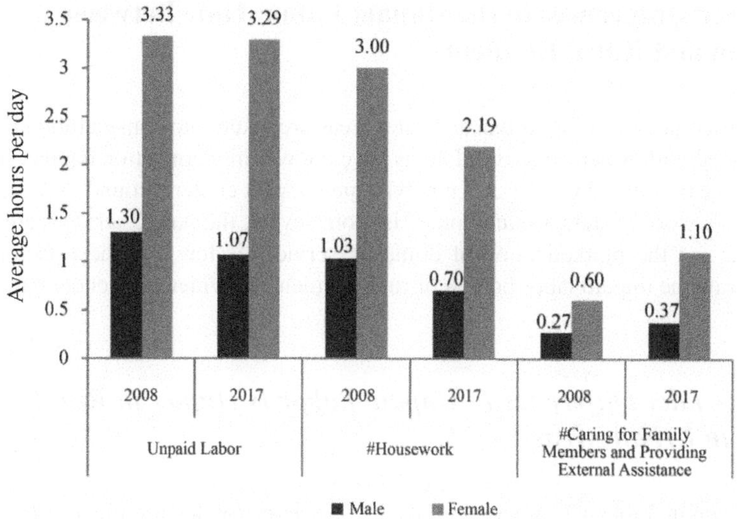

Fig. 4.2 Comparison of the average participation length of unpaid labor in 2008 and 2017

time became larger. The decrease in housework time for both men and women was mainly due to the development of the economy and the socialization of services. On the one hand, with the development of the service industry, the supply of various household and catering services has increased; on the other hand, residents' income has generally increased and they gradually seek alternative services to housework in the market. The average length of time spent by men and women caring for their families and providing external assistance has increased, mainly due to the increase in the average time spent caring for minors.[11] In other words, Chinese residents were willing to spend more time caring for their children, tutoring their homework, and accompanying them to study and read, etc. To sum up, there were gender differences in the impact of economic development and rising income levels on unpaid labor time with men's housework decreasing at a higher speed than women's, while men's participation length of caring for family members and providing external assistance increasing at a lower speed than that of women's. The ratio of women's to men's unpaid labor time increased from 2.56 in 2008 to 3.07 in 2017. The gender difference in unpaid labor has widened.

[11] Analysis of the types of unpaid labor reveals that housework and care of minors are the main activities that constitute unpaid labor.

Gender Differences in the Unpaid Labor Time Between Urban and Rural Residents

The differences between urban and rural areas are taken into consideration because compared with urban areas, rural areas have a lower modernization degree. In rural areas, the traditional gender concept that "men's work centers around outside, while women's work centers around home" is more severe, the public services are insufficient, and the marketization of domestic services is low. All these factors will aggravate the unpaid labor burden of rural women and widen the gender gap.

The Gender Difference in Unpaid Labor Is Higher in Rural than in Urban Areas

As shown in Table 4.3, in terms of average participation length, the average length of unpaid labor for urban women was 1.97 h per day more than that of men, and the average length of unpaid labor for rural women was 2.40 h per day more than that of men, of which, the average length of housework for urban women was 1.37 h per day more than that of men. The average length of housework for rural women was 1.59 h per day more than that of men. The average time spent by urban women caring for their families and providing external assistance was 0.60 h per day more than that of men, and the average time spent by rural women caring for their families and providing external assistance was 0.81 h per day more than that of men. The participation rate of urban women in unpaid labor was 32.8% points higher than that of men, and the participation rate of rural women in unpaid labor was 41.0% points higher than that of men, of which, the participation rate of urban women in housework was 33.8% points higher than that of men, and the participation rate of rural women in housework was 40.9% points higher than that of men. The participation rate of urban women in caring for family members and providing external assistance was 10.9% points higher than that of men, and the participation rate of rural women in caring for family members and providing external assistance was 13.0% points higher than that of men. It can be seen that the gender gap in unpaid labor is larger in rural than in urban areas, reflecting the relatively weaker bargaining power of rural women in housework, which leads to more unpaid labor for them.

The Gender Difference in Taking Care of Family Members and Relatives Is Higher in Rural Areas than in Urban Areas

As shown in Fig. 4.3, the average participation length spent by urban women caring for their families and relatives was 0.98 h per day, which was 0.61 h per day more than that of men. The average time spent by rural women caring for their families

Table 4.3 Basic situation of the time use of unpaid labor time by gender in urban and rural areas

		Urban		Rural	
		Male	Female	Male	Female
Unpaid labor	Average hours per day	1.14	3.11	1.05	3.45
	Participation rate (%)	43.0	75.8	38.6	79.6
	Participants' average hours per day	2.65	4.10	2.72	4.33
#Housework	Average hours per day	0.75	2.12	0.72	2.31
	Participation rate (%)	36.6	70.4	34.4	75.3
	Participants' average hours per day	2.05	3.01	2.09	3.07
#Caring for family members and providing external assistance	Average hours per day	0.39	0.99	0.33	1.14
	Participation rate (%)	12.3	23.2	8.3	21.3
	Participants' average hours per day	3.17	4.27	3.98	5.35

and relatives was 1.12 h per day, which was 0.84 h per day more than that of men. It can be seen that the gender difference in caring for family members and relatives was higher in rural than in urban areas, which might be partly due to the weak bargaining power of women in the household and more likely to be related to the traditional attitudes of residents, which were stronger in rural areas compared to urban areas, resulting in rural men spending less time in unpaid care than urban men and rural women spending more time in unpaid care than urban women.

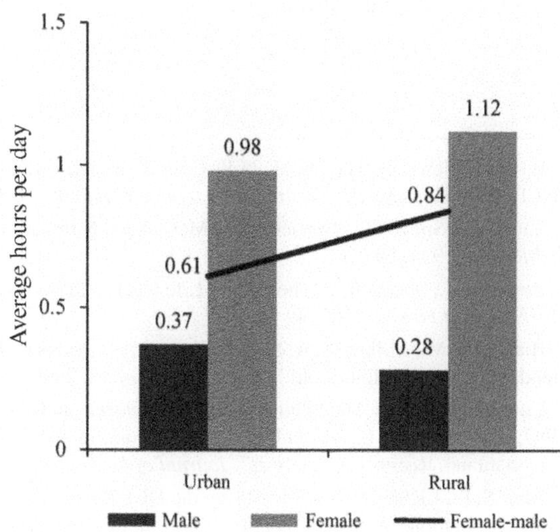

Fig. 4.3 Average time spent caring for family members and relatives in urban and rural areas

Gender Differences in Unpaid Labor Time Among Residents of Different Ages

This section discusses the distribution and gender differences in unpaid labor time for men and women at different stages of the life course from an age perspective. Many scholars have explored the time use of unpaid labor from a life-course perspective. Baxter (2008) studied the effects of marriage and parenthood transitions on couples' unpaid labor time and found that marriage and parenthood transitions had no significant effects on men's unpaid labor time, while women's unpaid labor time increased significantly after marriage and childbirth, and the gap in men's unpaid labor time input became larger.[12] Women spend more time on unpaid labor than men in different marital status, and this phenomenon is more obvious after marriage; married women spend the most time on unpaid labor compared with women in other marital status, while unmarried women spend the least; unmarried, cohabiting and married men spend very similar time on unpaid labor, but divorced or widowed men spend more time on unpaid labor than the unmarried, cohabiting and married men.[13] The type of unpaid labor in the household changes before and after the birth of a child.[14] Unpaid labor varies by the age of family members. The burden of unpaid labor increases for mothers, especially for those with preschool-age children.[15] However, the effect of preschool-age children on the father's housework time is uncertain.[16] Co-living teenage or adult children (especially daughters) who help share household chores may reduce the amount of unpaid labor time for both mothers and fathers.[17] Similarly, parents who live together or next to the married children and their spouses share unpaid labor and reduce their housework.[18] The order of these roles or events varies roughly with age. Therefore, the time input of residents' unpaid labor is different, and so are the gender differences.

---

[12] Baxter J., Hewitt B., Haynes M., "Life Course Transitions and Housework: Marriage, Parenthood, and Time on Housework", *Journal of Marriage & Family*, 2008, 70 (2).

[13] South S.J., Spitze G., "Housework in Marital and Nonmarital Households", *American Sociological Review*, 1994, 59 (3).

[14] Rexcroat C., Shehan C., "The Family Life Cycle and Spouses' Time in Housework", *Journal of Marriage and Family*, 1987, 49 (4).

[15] Bianchi S. M., Milkie M. A, Sayer L C, et al., "Is Anyone Doing the Housework? Trends in the Gender Division of Household Labor", *Social Forces*, 2000, 79 (1).

[16] Coltrane S., Family Man: Fatherhood, Housework, and Gender Equity. Oxford University Press, 1997; Kalleberg A. L., Rosenfeld R. A., "Work in the Family and in the Labor Market: A Crossnational, Reciprocal Analysis", *Journal of Marriage and the Family*, 1990, 52 (2).

[17] Blair S. L., Lichter D. T., "Measuring the Division of Household Labor: Gender Segregation of Housework among American Couples", *Journal of Family Issues*, 1991, 12 (1).

[18] Yang J., Short S., "Investigating China's 'Stalled Revolution': Husband and Wife Involvement in Housework in the PRC", Annual Meeting of Population Association of America, Philadelphia, PA. 2005.

The Participation Length of Unpaid Labor Is Greater for Women than for Men at All Ages

Figure 4.4 shows that the average time spent on unpaid labor is greater for women than for men, regardless of age. The largest difference between male and female unpaid labor time occurred at the age of 51–55 years old, with a difference of 3.26 h per day; the smallest difference occurred at the age of 16–20 years, with a difference of 0.34 h per day. In the age groups of 26–30 and 56–60 years old, there were two peaks of 3.82 h per day and 4.64 h per day in the average participation length of unpaid labor for women; the change in the average participation length of unpaid labor for men lagged behind that of women, with two peaks in the age groups of 31–35 and 61–70 years old, at 1.11 h per day and 1.84 h per day, respectively; the duration of unpaid labor for women aged 56–60 years old was greater than that of women aged 26–30 years old; the participation length of unpaid labor for older men aged 61–70 years old was greater than that of men aged 31–35 years old. Studies found that grandparents in urban families in which both the father and the mother worked took on almost all household chores, and it has become common in today's society for grandparents to take care of children and do housework (with older women still being the majority of housework) as a form of intergenerational support and intergenerational reciprocity.[19] Of course, the welfare of older women was severely curtailed.[20]

The reasons differ for the increase in the average participation length of unpaid labor for women between the age groups of 26–30 years old and 56–60 years old. Combining Figs. 4.5 and 4.6, it can be seen that the increase in unpaid labor hours for women at the age of 26–30 came mainly from caring for minors. According to data from the National Bureau of Statistics on fertility rates by age (sample survey of population), the highest fertility rates were observed among women of childbearing age of 25–29 years old from 2007 to 2015. The significant increase in unpaid labor among women aged 26–30 years old was mainly due to the care that accompanied the birth of a child. At the same time, there was an increase in care-giving by grandmothers aged 56–60 years old to grandchildren (1.3 h per day), but this was not the main reason for the increase in unpaid labor of older women aged 56–60. As shown in Fig. 4.4, the average participation length of housework for women gradually increased with growing age, reaching the maximum at the age of 56–60 years old (3.21 h per day) and then decreased. Thus, the increase in unpaid labor hours for women aged 56–60 years old came mainly from housework.

Although the average participation length of unpaid labor for men was smaller than that of women, its trend was very similar to that of women, except that after age 60, unlike women, the average participation length decreased significantly, but

---

[19] YiFei Shen, "Individualization and the Reconstruction of Family Structure", Doctoral Dissertation, Fudan University, 2010.

[20] Yanlan Tao, "Intergenerational Reciprocity or Inadequate Welfare—Intergenerational Exchange and Gender in Housework in Urban Families with Working Couple", *Journal of Chinese Women's Studies*, 2011 (4).

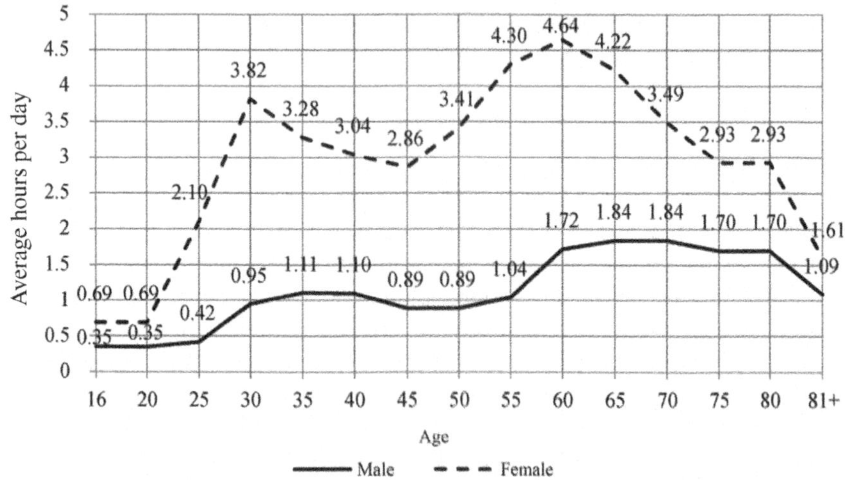

Fig. 4.4 Average participation length of unpaid labor for residents of different ages

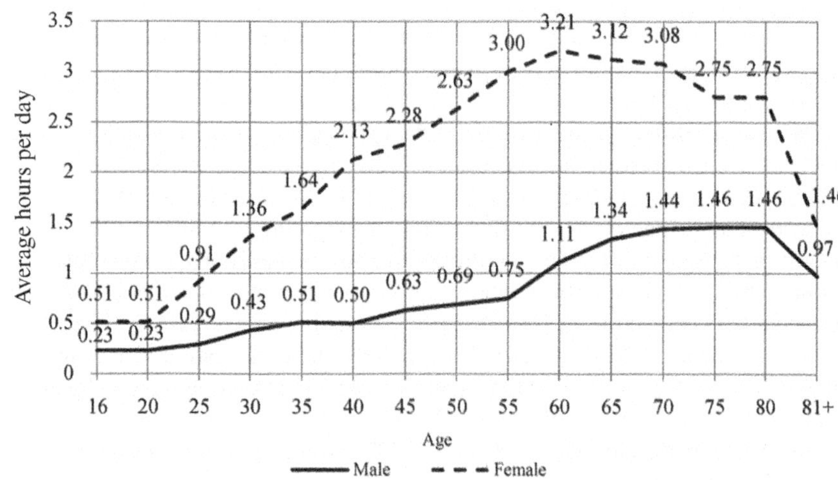

Fig. 4.5 Average participation length of housework for residents of different ages

remained stable until it became significantly lower after 80 years old. The change in the average time of unpaid labor for men lagged behind that of women, reaching the maximum at the age of 31–35 and 61–70 years old respectively (for women, it was at the age of 26–30 and 56–60 years old). Combining Fig. 4.5 with Fig. 4.6, it can be concluded that the two changes in men's unpaid labor time also came from the issue of childcare at birth, except that men joined childcare activities later than women, which was probably due to the fact that on average, men marry and have children at an age elder than women.

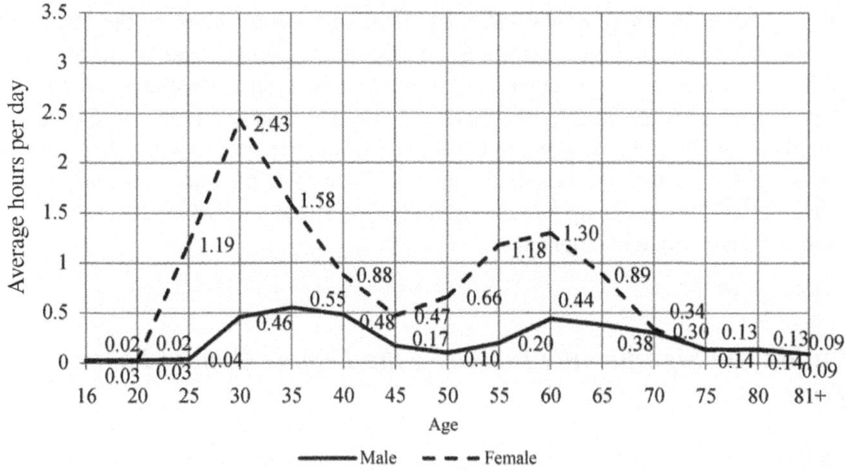

Fig. 4.6 Care of minors by residents of different ages

Marriage Has a Greater Impact on Women's Housework Time than Men's

Figure 4.5 shows that housework time increased with age until 60 years old for women, and 80 years old for males. The participation length decreased after 80 years old, which might be attributed to older age and poor health. Men and women had relatively less time for housework before the age of 20, with 0.23 h per day for men and 0.51 h per day for women. Women's housework time was close to 1 h per day at the age of 21–25 years old (the legal age of marriage for Chinese women is 20). Women's housework time increased with age, reaching a maximum of 3.21 h per day at the age of 56–60 years old, and decreased after 60 years old. Only at the age of 56–60 years (near the retirement age) did men reach more than 1 h of housework time per day. Before the age of 20, the difference between the housework time of men and women was relatively small, which was only 0.28 h per day. After the age of 20, the difference between the housework time of men and women gradually expanded, reaching more than 2 h per day in the age group of 51–60 years old, and then the difference narrowed and remained above 1 h. After the age of 80, both men's and women's housework time decreased. After 80 years old, the time spent on housework decreased for both men and women, but the difference between the two was still half an hour per day. At the same time, the data show that women aged 56–70 spent more time on housework than women in other age groups, and men aged 56 and above spent more time on housework than those in other age groups. Related studies have pointed out that age affects the distribution of housework time. For example, the increase in housework time with age (the survey respondents were

18–54 years old)[21] may be the effect of changing marital status on the one hand, as women's status and responsibilities change after marriage, and housework time gradually increased; on the other hand, it may be the effect of withdrawal from the labor market.[22] After quitting the labor market, they had relatively more time and would take on more housework. In China, retired elderly people will help their sons and daughters to take care of their families. Therefore, men and women aged 56 years old and above take up more household chores such as cooking, laundry, house cleaning, and simple maintenance.

Child Care Significantly Increases the Female Unpaid Labor Time

The birth of a child increases the unpaid labor time of men and women, and the change in unpaid labor time is more pronounced for women. Figure 4.6 shows that the average time spent caring for minors was 1.19 h per day, 2.43 h per day, and 1.58 h per day for women in the age groups of 21–25, 26–30, and 31–35 years old respectively. The average time spent by men caring for minors in the age groups of 21–25, 26–30 and 31–35 was 0.04, 0.46 and 0.55 h per day respectively. Mothers devoted more than 1 h per day to caring for minors than fathers. Mothers devoted almost two hours more than fathers, especially during the peak childbearing ages (26–29 years old for women). Women aged 51–60 years old took care of minors for more than one hour a day, and men aged 56–66 years old took care of minors for less than half an hour a day. Grandmothers invested 2.95 times more time than grandfathers. Mothers were the primary caregivers of minors, with grandmothers, fathers, and grandfathers playing a supportive role, among which grandmothers provided the primary assistance. The average time spent by mothers caring for minors was 1.13 h per day more than grandmothers and almost twice as much as that of grandmothers; grandmothers spent 0.75 and 0.86 h per day more than fathers and grandfathers caring for minors, respectively. As children grew older, the time spent by men and women in caring for them decreased, and the difference in time spent narrowed at the age of 40 to 50 years old for the caregiver, when the burden was relatively small. As for people aged 70 or above, there was almost no difference in the time spent between men and women caring for minors, and the values were small, which were less than 10 min per day. The energy allocation theory states that the allocation of time and energy determines the economic return of the individual in the labor market. The more time and energy women invest in the family, the less time and energy they invest in the labor

[21] Juhua Yang, "Gender Boundaries of Private Space from the Division of Housework", *Journal of Chinese Women's Studies*, 2006 (5).

[22] South S.J., Spitze G., "Housework in Marital and Nonmarital Households", *American Sociological Review*, 1994, 59 (3).

market, and the lower the economic returns to labor.[23] The constant accumulation of women's human capital was influenced by their going home to care for children, the interrupted work and insufficient input and inconsistency of employment. These may lead to a lack of work experience, vocational training and technical training. Women may have to choose jobs with little space for promotion, high flexibility, less energy consumption, shorter commute time and lower income, so that they can take care of the children and facilitate access to the labor market at any time. This phenomenon of women's income loss due to childbearing is called the Wage Penalty for Motherhood.[24] Having a child had caused a significant work-life conflict for women, resulting in lower employment rates,[25] with a 5–10% drop in income,[26] and a widening income gap in that of men. The Universal Two-Child Policy is a solution to the problem of insufficient labor supply and aging, and the adjustment of the fertility policy affects women as child-bearers. Under the existing social policy design and service planning system, it is worth exploring whether women will choose to have children since families have borne the cost of childbirth.

Care Deficit for the Elderly

In the sample of this chapter, 63% of the recipients of the caring for adults were the elderly (people aged 60 years old and above), so the situation of caring for adults roughly reflects the care-giving situation for the elderly. As shown in Fig. 4.7, the average participation length of caring for adults was small for both men and women, averaging about 4 min per day, with women taking 0.6 min more than men per day. The participation rates of caring for adults were 1.9% and 2.2% for men and women, respectively. As can be seen from Fig. 4.6, at around 30 years old, women spent an average of 2.43 h per day (about 146 min) caring for their own children. At around 60 years old, women spent 1.30 h per day (about 78 min) helping their sons and daughters care for their children (i.e., caring for their grandchildren), while men, despite not devoting as much time as women to caring for their children and grandchildren, still spent an average of 26 min per day at around 60 years old.

Figure 4.7 shows that both men and women spent less than 7 min a day caring for adults until the age of 60, and that there was a serious inequality in the so-called feedback mode,[27] with a "deficit" of care for the elderly. Figure 4.7 shows that men spent more time per day caring for adults than women until the age of 45. This

[23] JieXiao, "A Review of Sociological Research on Housework in China in the Past 20 Years", *Women's Academy at Shandong*, 2017 (3).

[24] Budig, M. J., England P., "The Wage Penalty for Motherhood", *American Sociological Review*, 2001, 66 (2).

[25] Yaowu Wu, "Stripping Income Effects and Substitution Effects—An Explanation of Changes in Urban Female Market Participation", *Studies in Labor Economics*, 2015 (4).

[26] Gough M., Noonan M., "A Review of the Motherhood Wage Penalty in the United States", *Sociology Compass*, 2013, 7 (4).

[27] The feedback mode refers to the two-way intergenerational care flow mode for families.

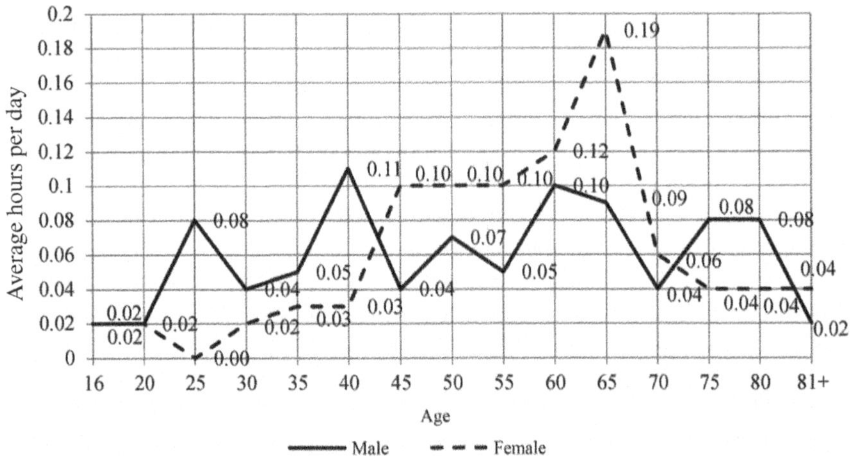

Fig. 4.7 Care of adults by residents of different ages

was probably due to the Chinese tradition of (a wife) living in the husband's home. Women spent more time taking care of adults at 45–70 years old than men did. The longest time taking care of adults appeared at 60–65 years old, which was 11 min on average every day. With the growth of age, women are liberated from taking care of minors and devote more time to taking care of adults (mostly their spouses or parents).

Gender Differences in Unpaid Labor Time Among Residents with Different Education Levels

This section explores how men and women with different education levels allocate their unpaid labor time and the differences between them. Education, as a resource, plays a large role in allocating housework. Increased education levels not only help reduce one's housework time by improving domestic living conditions and changing traditional attitudes, but also serve as bargaining capital within a household to help reduce one's housework time and the corresponding proportion. There is a significant gender difference in the effect of education levels on the allocation of housework time for couples.[28] For men, education positively affects the amount of time spent on housework, which means that husbands with higher education levels are more

[28] Junhui Hu, "Research on the Influencing Factors of Household Time Allocation", *Theoretic Observation*, 2014 (8).

likely to share housework with their wives.[29] Some studies have also concluded that women with more education do not significantly spend less time on unpaid labor.[30]

Unpaid Labor Time Is Longer for Women than Men with Different Education Levels

As shown in Fig. 4.8, the average participation length of unpaid labor for women is greater than that for men, regardless of education level. The difference in the average participation length of unpaid labor between women and men with different education levels was as high as 2.48 h per day and as low as 0.98 h per day. The higher the education level, the fewer time men and women spent on unpaid labor, and the smaller the difference between men's and women's unpaid labor time. As the education level increased, the average participation length of unpaid labor for women decreased, and the average participation length of unpaid labor for those who had not yet been to school was 1.42 h per day more than those who had a bachelor's degree and above. The overall trend in the average participation length of unpaid labor for men was also decreasing, with 0.18 h per day more for those who had not yet been to schools than for those with a bachelor's degree or above, but the change was no longer than that of women. The difference between women's and men's unpaid labor time varied in an inverted U shape as education level increased, from 2.22 h per day, 2.35 h per day and 2.48 h per day for people with an education level lower than high school, to 0.98 h per day for people with the bachelor's degree and above.

Education Reduces the Gender Gap in Housework

As Fig. 4.9 shows, the average participation length of housework for men and women gradually decreases as the education level increases. On average, the unschooled female population spent 1.68 h per day more on unpaid work than those with a bachelor's degree and above. The average participation length of housework for men fluctuated with the increase in education level, but the overall trend was decreasing, and the average participation length of housework for those who did not attend school was 0.35 h per day more than those with bachelor's degrees and above. The effect of education level on women was much greater than that on men. Men had fewer hours of housework regardless of their education level, while women's participation length of housework decreased significantly with the increase in education levels.

[29] Hongqin Chang, Xiaoyuan Dong, Fiona MacPhail, "The Impact of Economic Development on Gender Patterns of Household Time Allocation in Chinese Rural Areas", *Chinese Rural Economy*, 2009 (12).

[30] Xiaoyan Yuan, Lei Shi, "Research on the Impact of Education Levels on Female Labor Time Allocation", *Shanghai Journal of Economics*, 2017 (6).

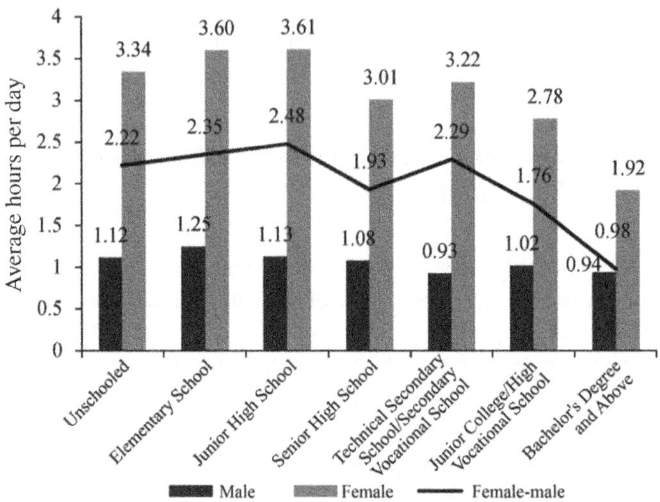

Fig. 4.8 Unpaid labor of residents with different education levels

The difference in housework time between women and men gradually narrowed with increasing education, ranging from 1.74 h per day for those unschooled to 0.41 h per day for those with a bachelor's degree and above. From the perspective of the Relative Resources Theory, structural resources (education, occupation, and income) influence the ability to negotiate between couples and are one of the main determinants of the allocation of housework.[31] As housework is boring and unrewarding, the one with more resources tends to invest less in housework or even avoid it.[32] Between spouses, the one with a higher education level, better career reputation and more income has the stronger negotiation ability and the more dominant power in the allocation of housework.[33] The more educated they are, the more likely they are to have access to better job opportunities and are more willing to buy housework services. In addition, those with higher education levels have stronger gender equality concepts. For example, women demand that the allocation of housework be equal, and husbands are willing to share more of the housework, making the allocation of housework within the family more equal.[34]

[31] Juhua Yang, "Gender Boundaries of Private Space from the Division of Housework", *Journal of Chinese Women's Studies*, 2006 (5).

[32] Blair S. L., Lichter D. T., "Measuring the Division of Household Labor: Gender Segregation of Housework among American Couples", *Journal of Family Issues*, 1991, 12 (1); Huber J., Spitze G. D., "Sex Stratification: Children Housework and Jobs", *New York N*, 1983, 46 (1).

[33] Brines J., "Economic Dependency, Gender, and the Division of Labor at home", *American Journal of Sociology*, 1994, 100 (3): 652–688.

[34] Juhua Yang, "Gender Boundaries of Private Space from the Division of Housework", *Journal of Chinese Women's Studies*, 2006 (5).

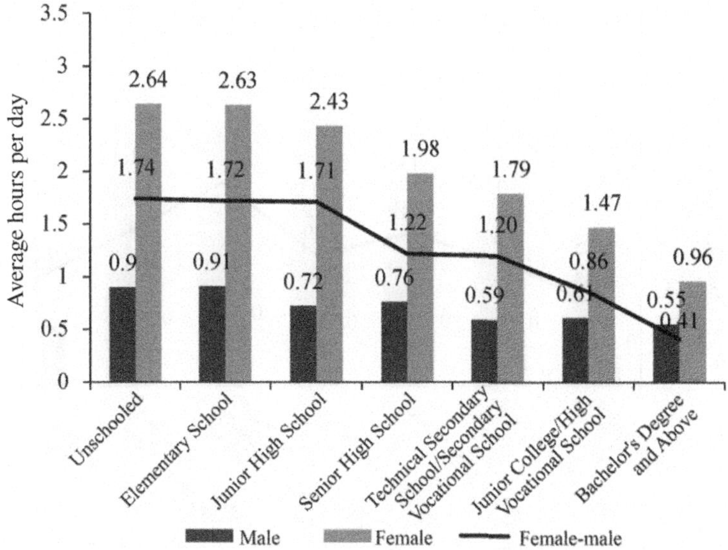

Fig. 4.9 Housework of residents with different education levels

Highly Educated Mothers Spend More Time Caring for Their Children

Figure 4.10 shows that the average time spent caring for minors increased in an inverted U-shape for women as their education level increased, and increased for men overall. Both men and women who had never been to school spent the least amount of time caring for minors, and the amount of time spent by both men and women increased as their education level increased. The difference in the average time spent caring for minors between men and women showed an inverted U-shape as education level increased, with higher education levels resulting in smaller differences in the time spent caring for minors. Studies have pointed out that parents' time investment in children is of great importance to their human capital development, and that parents who have received more education spend more time with their children. That is, the more educated parents spend more time feeding and nursing their children, putting them to bed, reading books to them, teaching them moral lessons, tutoring them with homework, and playing games with them. Moreover, children of more educated parents preferred the company of their parents, and these parents invested their time more efficiently.[35] Parents with higher education levels were more conducive to their children's development in terms of their ability and concept of investing in their children's education.

[35] Guryan J., Hurst E., Kearney M., "Parental Education and Parental Time with Children", *Journal of Economic Perspectives*, 2008, 22 (3).

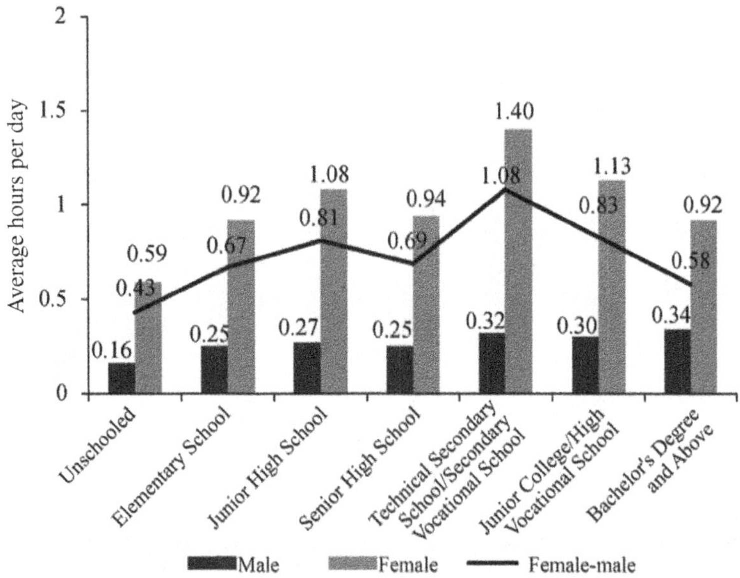

Fig. 4.10 Care of minors by residents of different education levels

Gender Differences in Unpaid Labor Time of Residents of Different Income Levels

This section explores how men and women at different household income levels allocate their unpaid labor time and the differences between them. The New Family Economics argues that the wage of a worker in the market is the opportunity cost of performing housework within the household.[36] People with higher incomes face higher opportunity costs of unpaid labor, so they are less inclined to do unpaid labor. Related studies have been conducted, more from the theory of relative resources, believing that the party with higher income can do less housework and continuously reduce his or her own housework time through the relatively increasing income.[37] However, influenced by traditional gender concepts, when women's relative incomes exceed a certain range, wives will instead increase their housework time as their income increases relatively.[38]

In this section, all sample households were divided into five sample groups: low-income, lower-income, middle-income, higher-income, and high-income, based on

[36] Junhui Hu, "The Influence of Occupation on the Choice of Labor Time Allocation: The Example of Housework Time", *Population and Development*, 2015 (2).

[37] Bittman M., England P., Sayer L., et al., "When does Gender Trump Money? Bargaining and Time in Household Work", *American Journal of Sociology*, 2003, 109 (1).

[38] Jia Yu, "Gender Concepts, Modernization and Women's Housework Time", *Society*, 2014 (2).

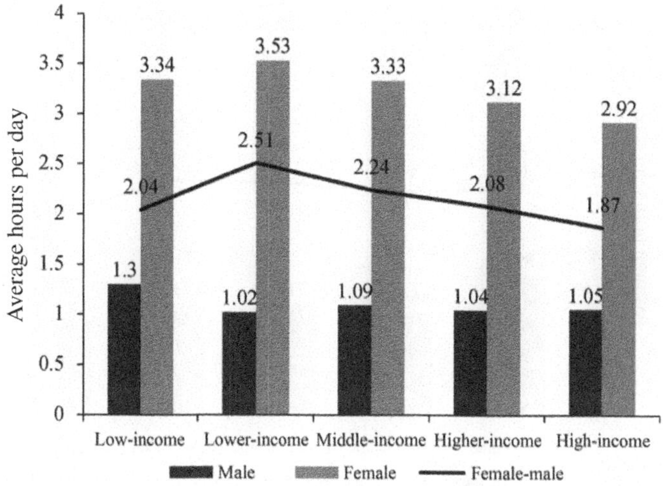

Fig. 4.11 The average participation length of unpaid labor across different income levels

the quintiles of annual provincial per capita household income from the lowest to the highest.

The Gender Gap Shows an Inverted U-shape with Income

As shown in Fig. 4.11, the overall trend shows an inverted U-shaped change in women's unpaid labor time and a gradual decrease in men's unpaid labor time as income increases. The average participation length of unpaid labor for men decreased from 1.30 h per day to 1.05 h per day, a decrease of 19.2%; the average participation length of unpaid labor for women decreased from 3.34 h per day to 2.92 h per day, a decrease of 12.6%, and the decrease rate for women was smaller than that for men. From the difference in the average participation length of unpaid labor between men and women, the gender difference decreased with the increase in income, and the gender difference in unpaid labor was the smallest in the high-income group.

Low-Income People Have a Heavier Burden of Housework

Figure 4.12 shows that the average participation length of housework for low-income women is higher than other types including the national average level. This is also the case for low-income men. The average participation length of housework for low-income women was 2.33 h per day, while that for low-income men was 0.89 h per day. The gender difference in average housework time decreased with the increase

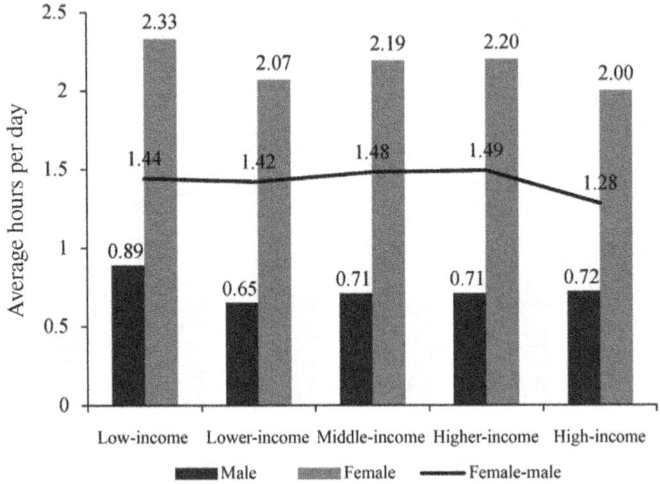

Fig. 4.12 Average participation length of house-work by different income levels

in income, and the gender difference in the high-income group was the smallest. It can be seen that housework was more onerous for low-income people and easier for high-income people, because high-income households can reduce the burden of housework by purchasing services.

The Time Spent by Women Caring for Family Members and Relatives Showed an Inverted U-shape with Income

Figure 4.13 shows that the average participation time spent caring for family members and relatives varies little across income levels, with 0.35 h per day for low-income men and 0.32 h per day for high-income men, a difference of fewer than 2 min per day. Looking at the different income groups, the average participation length of time spent caring for family members and relatives was relatively higher for lower and middle-income women. The difference in the average time spent caring for family members and relatives between men and women showed an inverted U-shape with increasing income, and the gender difference in unpaid care-giving was the smallest among the high-income group.

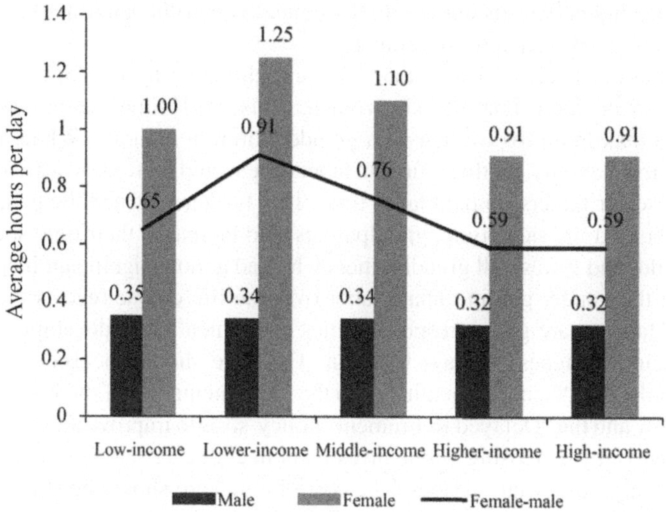

Fig. 4.13 Average participation length of caring for family members and relatives by different income levels

Summary

Using data from the 2017 Chinese Time Use Survey, this chapter analyzes the gender differences in unpaid labor time of residents in urban and rural areas, across ages, with different education levels, and income levels. The data show that women's unpaid labor time was much higher than that of men, about 2.95 times the average participation length of men's unpaid labor. The gender difference in unpaid labor was not only in the average participation length, but also in the flexibility of the type of activities performed. Daily housework and caring for minors, which differed significantly between men and women, were both activities with less time flexibility and more solidified in their schedules, which had a more pronounced impact on work and life. From 2008 to 2017, unpaid labor time had decreased for both men and women, the average time spent caring for family members had increased for women, and the overall gender ratio of unpaid labor time had become larger.

From an urban–rural perspective, the average time spent on unpaid labor was 2.40 h per day more for women than men in rural areas, and 1.97 h per day more for women than men in towns, with the gender difference in unpaid labor higher in rural areas than in towns; the average time spent on caring for family members and relatives was 0.84 h per day more for women than for men in rural areas, and 0.61 h per day more for women than for men in urban areas. The gender difference in caring for family members and relatives was also higher in rural than in urban areas. In order to reduce the burden of housework on rural women and narrow the gap between urban and rural areas, the government can increase the provision of public services to rural areas, raise rural income levels, promote the development of rural service industries, encourage rural women to enter the labor market, and raise awareness of gender equality in rural areas.

From the perspective of age, marriage and childcare have a bigger impact on women than on men. For married women, housework time increased with age, reaching a maximum for women with grandchildren in a family. When there were newborns in the family, mothers' unpaid labor time would increase to a greater extent, while not so for fathers' unpaid labor time. This further widened the gender gap in unpaid labor. At the same time, grandparents also increased their time spent caring for the child, and it was still grandmothers who had a more significant increase. The change in the gender gap in unpaid labor over the life course reveals the negative impact of family care-giving responsibilities on women's own development, which affects their willingness to have children. The state should incorporate the basic national policy of "Gender Equality" into the implementation of the Universal Two-Child Policy and the "Delayed Retirement" policy, so as to improve the existing social service system by increasing public investment in childcare services, and promoting the equalization of social services. The cost of childcare should be shared between society and families to distribute care responsibilities more equally between men and women within the family.[39]

From an educational perspective, education helps to reduce the burden of housework and narrow the gender gap. Education increases women's negotiating power in the household and reduces women's burden of housework. In addition, education can change traditional gender concepts and encourage men to share household chores and family care. Therefore, based on the full universalization of nine-year compulsory education, the state should further promote the popularization of higher education, establish a basic public education service system, narrow the education gap between urban and rural areas, and improve the national student financial aid system so that the education rights of rural girls can be better protected.

From an income perspective, the average participation length of unpaid labor for low-income men and women is greater than those of middle and high income earners, and low-income earners are more likely to face the "time and financial" burdens than better-off households. They do not have the financial means to purchase social services or modern appliances, so they spend more time on household chores, which in turn takes away from their paid labor time. At the same time, low-income people tend to have a low level of education and spend less quality time with their children despite spending more time on unpaid labor; they leave their children in the care of their grandparents (left-behind children) in order to improve their family's economic situation, causing more social problems. Society should pay more attention to this group and provide targeted social welfare policies to help them reduce the pressure of life and improve the quality of life.

---

[39] Jie Xiao, "How Big Is the Income Penalty Effect of Childbirth—A Study Based on the Income Distribution of Married Women", *Journal of Southeast University (Philosophy and Social Science)*, 2017 (3).

Chapter 5
Women Returning to the Family

The traditional gender division of labor within the family determines the status of couples in the family and society. In most countries around the world, the traditional gender division of labor is that "men's work centers around outside, while women's work centers around home", i.e., men are mainly responsible for paid market labor, while women are mainly responsible for unpaid labor such as housework and care-giving. With the progress in social development and gender equality, more and more women are entering the labor market, but unpaid labor is still performed mainly by women. China is no exception.[1] Unpaid labor is critical to family welfare, and because there is no direct monetary return for these activities, women's contributions to the family are severely undervalued. The burden of family care-giving reduces women's employment opportunities and income, increases women's economic dependence on men, and weakens women's bargaining power within the family.[2] The double burden of work and family makes women more likely than men to fall into "time poverty" and not have enough time to rest and enjoy leisure time, which limits women's development.[3] It can be concluded that the unequal allocation of labor time within the family is one of the important causes of gender inequality.

The gender division of labor within households is not only about social equity, but also has important implications for economic growth and population structure. McKinsey Global Institute estimates that there is a gender gap in economic participation rates in many countries around the world due to factors such as traditional gender role positioning and gender discrimination, and that if women's economic participation could be raised to the level of men's, China's GDP would increase by

[1] Juhua Yang, "Gender Differences in Time-use: An Analysis of its Changing Trends and Characteristics from 1990 to 2010", *Population & Economics*, 2014 (5); Chi Zhang, "Gender Difference in Total Working Hours and Its Influencing Factors: Based on Basic Survey Data of Social Life in Japan", Master Dissertation, Jinan University, 2016.

[2] Boserup Ester, "Women's Role in Economic Development", *American Journal of Agricultural Economics*, 1970, 53 (3).

[3] Liangshu Qi, Xiao-yuan Dong, "Gender, Low-paid Status, and Time Poverty in Urban China", *Feminist Economics*, 2018, 24 (2).

F. Du et al., *Chinese People's Time Use and Their Quality of Life*,
https://doi.org/10.1007/978-981-99-5526-8_5

an additional US$2.5 trillion in 2025, and global GDP would increase by an additional US$28 trillion over the same period.[4] Gender equality in the economic sector (paid labor) is closely related to how unpaid labor time is distributed between the sexes within the household: it is impossible to achieve equal economic participation of women and men if the majority of household care is performed by women, because the time and energy of human are limited. Faced with the "double pressure" of work and family, many women will have to make a choice between the two. Many developed countries advocate gender equality in education and labor markets, but their social policies still maintain the traditional gender division of labor, so many women choose not to marry or have children in the face of the constraints on personal development imposed by family care.[5] In turn, low fertility accelerates population aging and labor shortages, constraining sustainable economic development.

Studies in developed countries show that gender differences in the allocation of labor time within households are positively correlated with the degree of gender equality. In some Nordic countries, economic development has been accompanied by institutional changes to traditional gender relations. On the one hand, the state has promoted gender equality in the labor market through legislation against gender discrimination and equal pay for equal work between men and women; on the other hand, it has encouraged men and women to share family care by providing shared maternity and parental leave, increasing investment in childcare institutions and preschool education, and promoting "family-friendly" work arrangements to reduce women's burden of unpaid work and work-family conflict. In these countries, not only are labor participation rates and gender wage gaps smaller, but the gender gap in the division of paid and unpaid labor and total labor time within households are also smaller, and the fertility rates are relatively high.[6] In Southern European countries such as Italy and Greece, as well as East Asian countries such as Japan and Korea, economic growth has not fundamentally changed the traditional pattern of "men's work centers around outside, while women's work centers around home", and social policies and family taxation patterns are basically designed according to the traditional gender division of labor. As a result, gender differences and inequalities within households and in the labor market are relatively large in these countries, and fertility rates are relatively low.[7]

Achieving gender equality is a fundamental national policy in China. The *United Nations 2030 Agenda for Sustainable Development* includes "achieving gender equality and empowering all women and girls" as one of the 17 Sustainable Development Goals, and proposes to recognize the value of unpaid domestic and care work

---

[4] McKinsey Global Institute, "The Power of Parity: How Advancing Women's Equality Can Add $12 Trillion to Global Growth", 2015.

[5] Peter McDonald, "Gender Equity, Social Institutions and the Future of Fertility", *Journal of Population Research*, 2000, 17 (1).

[6] Francesca Bettio, Janneke Plantenga, "Comparing Care Regimes in Europe", *Feminist Economics*, 2004, 10 (1).

[7] Mary C. Briton, Xiana Bueno Garcia, Olah Livia Sz, et al., "Postindustrial Fertility Ideals, Intentions, and Gender Inequality: A Comparative Qualitative Analysis", *Population and Development Review*, 2018, 44 (2).

and achieve gender equality by promoting infrastructure development, increasing public services, and encouraging family members to share the burden of unpaid labor more equally.

This chapter uses data from the 2008 and 2017 Chinese Time Use Survey. It analyzes the household gender division of labor changes in China and compares them with some developed and transitional countries. Understanding the changing trends in the household gender division of labor in China is of great practical significance for recognizing the disadvantaged position of women in the household and labor market, formulating economic and social policies that are conducive to the joint development of both sexes, implementing the basic state policy of gender equality, and achieving the 2030 Sustainable Development Goals.

Institutional Changes

In traditional Chinese society, the traditional concept of "men's work centers around outside, while women's work centers around home" has profoundly impacted women's low status. Since the founding of the People's Republic of China, the state has made women's participation in social production a core initiative to improve the status of women by providing paid maternity leave and subsidized childcare and kindergartens to ease the care burden of women and increase their labor force participation rate. Most Chinese women enter the workforce right after leaving school, working full-time like men. The family where both the husband and the wife work is the basic mode for Chinese families. While "women hold up half the sky" in the workplace, society still regards caring for the family as a "natural duty" for women, who carry the double burden of work and family.

Since the reform and opening-up, the state has made gender equality a basic state policy and has formulated a series of new policies and regulations to guarantee that women and men have the same political, economic and social rights. The rapid economic growth, industrialization and urbanization, and the development of the service industry have provided new jobs for women. The increase in women's education level has created conditions for narrowing the gender income gap. At the same time, the increase in household income, the development of the service industry market, and the promotion of labor-saving appliances have reduced the burden of women's housework.

The reform and opening-up has created new opportunities and challenges for Chinese women. There are even calls for "women to return to the family" in society. The second and third surveys on the social status of Chinese women show that the proportion of men who agree with the view that "men should focus on their careers and women should focus on their families" increased from 53.9 to 61.6% and from 50.4 to 54.8% between 2000 and 2010. The reform of state-owned enterprises and the expansion of the private and informal sectors have made it more difficult to monitor and implement labor laws and regulations to protect women's rights and interests. In the face of fierce market competition, some employers are reluctant to recruit women of marriage and childbearing age, especially after launching the Universal Two-Child Policy in 2016, women of childbearing age are subject to various overt and covert discrimination in looking for jobs.[8] Many women in the private and informal sectors have to withdraw from the labor market after having children because they do not have maternity insurance and are not entitled to maternity leave.[9]

Since the reform and opening up, social welfare policies were once positioned in such a way that "caring for children and the elderly is a private matter for the family". The reform of the welfare system has led to a decline in the supply of public childcare services, and the absence of institutional childcare services for 0–2-year-olds has had a negative impact on the employment of urban mothers with preschool-aged children.[10] At the same time, the high cost of childcare reduces the net benefits of employment for mothers, thereby reducing their willingness to take up employment, especially for those working in the low-income sectors.[11] The scarcity of childcare services has led many grandparents to help their sons and daughters care for the grandchildren, which also reduces labor force participation and non-farm employment among grandparents (mainly grandmothers) who are still of employment age (45–64 years old).[12] With increasing competition in the labor market and the intensifying differentiation in social classes, Chinese parents have become more "anxious" about their children's education than ever before, and families have increased their investment in early childcare and education so that their children do not lose out at the starting line; children are mainly taken care of by mothers, which further increases the unpaid labor burden of married women. The decline in the labor force participation rate of married women has eroded the family model that both parents work in China. This has also increased the economic pressure on married men to work longer hours and overtime to increase their income and cover household expenses. All of these changes affect the gender division of paid and unpaid labor within Chinese households.

---

[8] Desheng Lai, et al., "2016 China Labor Market Development Report: Female Employment in the Process of Gender Equalization", Beijing Normal University Publishing House, 2017: 147–158.

[9] Nan Jia, Xiao-yuan Dong, Yue-ping Song, "Paid Maternity Leave and Breastfeeding in Urban China", *Feminist Economics*, 2018, 24 (2).

[10] Fenglian Du, Xiao-yuan Dong, "Women's Employment and Childcare Choices in Urban China during the Economic Transition", *Economic Development and Cultural Change*, 2013, 62 (1).

[11] Yueping Song, Xiao-yuan Dong, "Childcare Costs and Migrant and Local Mothers' Labor Force Participation in Urban China", *Feminist Economics*, 2018, 24 (2).

[12] Fenglian Du, Yingyu Zhang, Xiaoyuan Dong, "The Impact of Child Care Practices on the Labor Force Participation Rate of Women in Urban China", *World Economics Papers*, 2018 (3); Yafeng Wang, Chuanchuan Zhang, "Gender Inequalities in Labor Market Outcomes of Informal Caregivers near Retirement Age in Urban China", *Feminist Economics*, 2018, 24 (2).

Women's Choice? From "Double Pressure" to "Return to the Family"

The data used in this section come from the 2008 Chinese Time Use Survey by the National Bureau of Statistics and the 2017 Chinese Time Use Survey by Inner Mongolia University. To ensure the comparability of data, the sample in this section includes only 10 provinces and cities covered by both surveys: Beijing, Hebei, Heilongjiang, Zhejiang, Anhui, Henan, Guangdong, Sichuan, Yunnan, and Gansu. The sample focuses on residents aged 22–64 who are married and living with their spouses. The sample does not include adult children and their spouses and elderly parents living with the head of the household because spousal relationships cannot be identified. There were 12,507 households in the 2008 sample and a total of 2008 households in the 2017 sample.

We used the female-to-male time ratio as a measure of the gender gap.[13] If the ratio is equal to 1, there is no difference; if the ratio is greater than 1 or less than 1, there is a difference. Unlike the gender time gap, the gender time ratio removes the effect of the base. For example, the average daily unpaid labor time for women in household A is 3 h and for men is 1 h, and the gender time gap is 2 h; the average daily unpaid labor time for women in household is 1.5 h and for men is 0.5 h, and the gender time gap is 1 h. We say that both households have 3 times more unpaid labor hours for women than for men, with the same gender time ratio of 3 and the same gender difference.

Overall Situation

Before analyzing the changes in the time use of married men (husbands) and married women (wives) within households, we look at the changes in their labor force participation rates from 2008 to 2017. Overall, the labor force participation rate of Chinese residents remained high, but there were clear gender differences. In 2008, the labor force participation rate increased to 88.7% for men and 78.9% for women; in 2017, the labor force participation rate was 89.9% for men and decreased to 74.2% for women. The gap between female and male labor force participation rates rose from 9.8% points to 15.7% points.

As shown in Fig. 5.1, the labor force participation rate of Chinese residents shows a trend of rising and then falling as age grows. If analyzed by gender, the labor force participation rate for men increased slightly in 2017 compared with 2008, but the lines of labor force participation rates were very close in both years, and there was no significant separation throughout the working age group. The labor force participation rate for women, on the other hand, differed significantly in two age groups: first, for women aged 22–38 years old, the labor force participation rate in

[13] This approach is common in international literature. See the *World Economic Forum's Global Gender Gap Report 2017.*

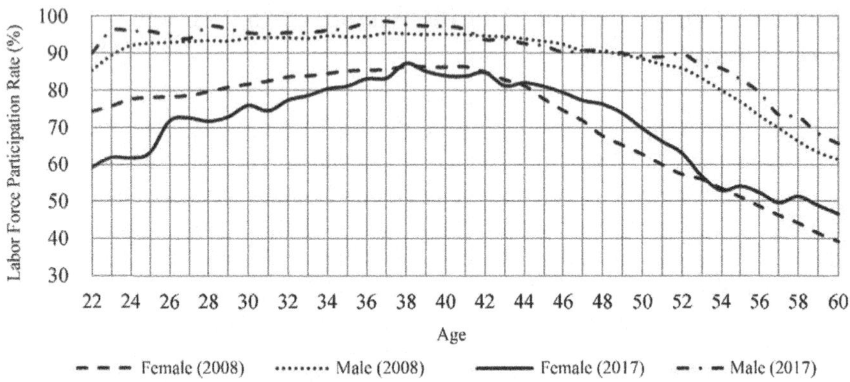

Fig. 5.1 Labor force participation rate of residents by age. *Source* The 2008 and 2017 Chinese Time Use Survey

2017 was significantly lower than that in 2008; second, for women aged 45–60 years old, the labor force participation rate was significantly higher than that in 2008, which reflected the impact of China's Universal Two-Child Policy and the delayed retirement of women.

As shown in Fig. 5.2, the age of children has a greater impact on female labor force participation rates, with the rates declining more in households with preschool and elementary school children than they did nine years ago, to which Figs. 5.1 and 5.2 correspond the findings for women aged 22–38 years old. The labor force participation rate for women with children aged 0–2 years old declined from 72.4% in 2008 to 61.4% in 2017, a decline of 11% points; for women with children aged 3–6 years old, the labor force participation rate declined from 80.6% in 2008 to 68.8% in 2017. The labor force participation rate for women with children aged 7–12 years old declined by 3.7% points, from 81.7% in 2008 to 78.0% in 2017. In contrast, the labor force participation rate for women without children aged 0–18 years old at home increased by 3.2% points from 81.0% in 2008 to 84.2% in 2017.

Following the withdrawal of some women of childbearing age from the labor market, the gender income gap has narrowed, with the ratio of female to male wages rising from 0.72 to 0.79, reflecting the change in net demand in China's labor market. On the one hand, after the outbreak of the international financial crisis in 2008, China's economic growth model shifted from export-oriented to domestic demand-driven, thus promoting the rapid development of the service sector and increasing the demand for female labor; on the other hand, the withdrawal of some women of childbearing age from the labor market reduced labor supply, and these changes caused female income to rise faster than male income, thus narrowing the gender income gap.

Table 5.1 reports selected gender time use within Chinese households. There are obvious gender differences in the division of labor within Chinese households: women have less paid labor time than men, more unpaid labor time than men, more total labor time than men, and less leisure time than men. From 2008 to 2017, paid

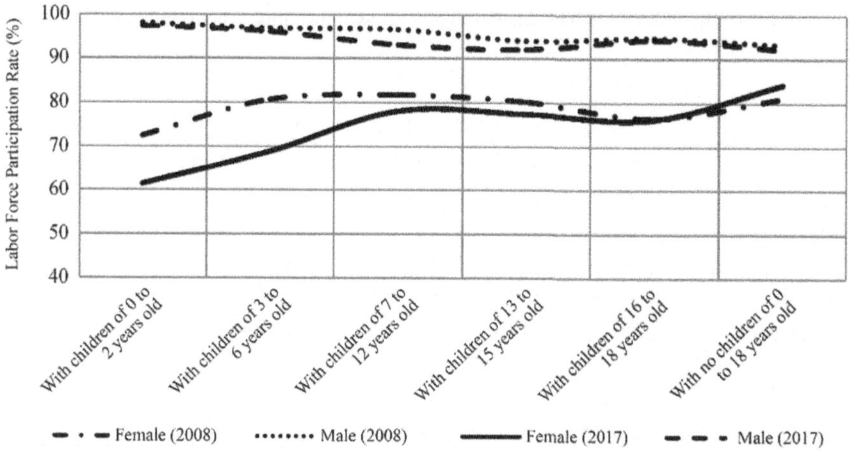

Fig. 5.2 Labor force participation rates of Chinese residents aged 22–49 by household structure. *Note* Since detailed information on the household structure is not available from the 2008 Chinese Time Use Survey, the data in 2008 are from the 2008 CHIP. *Source* The 2008 CHIP and 2017 Chinese Time Use Survey

labor time increased for both men and women, but men increased more than women, and the time ratio of female-to-male paid labor decreased from 0.73 to 0.71. At the same time, unpaid work time decreased for both men and women, with women's unpaid work time decreasing less than men's, and the ratio of female-to-male unpaid labor time increased from 2.68 in 2008 to 3.32 in 2017. The decrease in unpaid labor time was mainly due to the decrease in housework time and the increase in time spent caring for family members instead. Compared to 2008, total labor time increased for men and decreased slightly for women, the gender gap in total labor time decreased from 0.81 to 0.44 h per day, and the ratio of total labor time decreased from 1.10 to 1.05. As the distribution of total labor time became more even, the distribution of time for activities such as leisure and self-care also became more even between genders.

Table 5.2 reports the time use of households where both spouses were employed. Women in double-income households bear the double burden of work and family, and usually, their total labor time is longer than that of men. As can be seen from Table 5.2, both in 2008 and 2017, double-income households featured that women had less paid labor time than men, more unpaid labor time than men, more total labor time than men, and less leisure time than men. From 2008 to 2017, both men's and women's paid labor time increased (by 0.82 h per day for men and 0.75 h per day for women), with a somewhat larger increase in paid labor hours for women relative to their respective bases; thus, the ratio of paid labor hours for women to men increased slightly. As in the national aggregate, both men and women in double-income households saw a decrease in unpaid labor hours (0.37 h per day for men and 0.74 h per day for women), with women's unpaid labor hours decreasing from 2.26 h per day more than men to 1.89 h per day, while the ratio of women's to men's

Table 5.1 Gender differences and changes in time use within Chinese households

Unit: hours/day

	2008			2017		
	Male	Female	Female/male	Male	Female	Female/male
Paid labor	6.66	4.89	0.73	7.34	5.20	0.71
Unpaid labor[a]	1.54	4.13	2.68	1.11	3.68	3.32
#Housework	1.16	3.40	2.93	0.72	2.53	3.51
#Care for family members	0.32	0.67	2.09	0.39	1.15	2.95
Total labor	8.20	9.01	1.10	8.45	8.89	1.05
Leisure	4.09	3.47	0.85	4.05	3.56	0.88
Self-care	11.65	11.45	0.98	11.40	11.44	1.00
Labor force participation rate[b] (%)	88.7	78.9	−9.8	89.9	74.2	−15.7
Monthly labor income (Yuan)	1642	1182	0.72	3951	3102	0.79
Observed value	12,507	12,507		2008	2008	

Note [a] Unpaid labor includes housework, caring for family members, etc., same as the table below. [b] Gender labor participation rate gap is the labor participation rate of women minus the labor participation rate of men, same as the table below

Source The 2008 and 2017 Chinese Time Use Survey

unpaid labor hours increased from 2.76 to 3.08. Compared with 2008, the total labor time of men increased by 0.45 h per day, while the total labor time of women did not change; therefore, the total labor time of women decreased from 0.89 h per day more than men to only 0.44 h per day more than men, and the ratio of total labor time decreased from 1.10 to 1.05. The total labor time of double-income households was more equally distributed, and this change was mainly brought about by the decrease in the unpaid labor time of women, rather than by a more equal distribution of the unpaid labor burden.

Gender Differences in the Time Use Within Urban and Rural Households

There are significant differences in the work and lifestyle of urban and rural residents, so this subsection analyzes gender differences of time use in households in urban and rural areas. Table 5.3 reports the status and trends of time use of urban and rural households.

First of all, the data in urban areas have the same trend as the national change. The urban male labor participation rate increased from 82.9 to 86.9% from 2008 to 2017,

Table 5.2 Gender differences and changes in time use within double-income households in China

Unit: hours/day

	2008			2017		
	Male	Female	Female/male	Male	Female	Female/male
Paid labor	7.62	6.24	0.82	8.44	6.99	0.83
Unpaid labor	1.28	3.54	2.76	0.91	2.80	3.08
#Housework	0.97	3.00	3.10	0.64	2.07	3.23
#Care for family members	0.26	0.50	1.91	0.27	0.72	2.67
Total labor	8.90	9.79	1.10	9.35	9.79	1.05
Leisure	3.50	2.87	0.82	3.35	2.88	0.86
Self-care	11.54	11.28	0.98	11.20	11.22	1.00
Monthly labor income (Yuan)	1642	1182	0.72	4278	3203	0.75
Observed value	9257	9257		1147	1147	

Source The 2008 and 2017 Chinese Time Use Surveys

and the female labor participation rate decreased from 69.8 to 67.1%, and the gender labor participation rate difference expanded from 13.1 to 19.8% points; however, the gender income gap narrowed, with the female-to-male wage ratio rising from 0.73 to 0.77. The widening gender labor force participation rate gap affects the division of labor within urban households. As shown in Table 5.3, the paid labor hours of both men and women in urban households increased and the unpaid labor hours decreased, but the gender gap between the two types of labor widened. While men's daily paid labor hours were on average 1.39 h more than women's in 2008, this figure expanded to 2.29 h in 2017, and the ratio of women's to men's paid labor hours decreased from 0.74 to 0.68. The gender difference in unpaid labor hours widened slightly (from 2.33 to 2.36 h per day), and the ratio of unpaid labor hours for women to men increased from 2.22 to 2.84. These changes brought about a change in the gender difference in total labor hours, with women's total labor hours being 0.93 h per day more than men's in 2008, and in 2017 women's total labor time was 0.07 h per day more than that of men. The ratio of total female to male labor time decreased from 1.13 to 1.01, and the distribution of leisure time between men and women became more even as a result. Although the widening gender gap in paid labor has narrowed the gender gap in total labor time to some extent, women's contribution to household income has decreased, with women's share of total household income decreasing from 40% in 2008 to 37.3%, and women's economic dependence has increased.[14]

The second part of Table 5.3 reports the time use of rural households. Unlike the trend of change in urban areas, not only the labor force participation rate of

[14] The author only calculated the share of women in total household labor income in urban households, because the contribution of individuals cannot be quantified for rural household labor income, which includes the household agricultural business income.

Table 5.3 Gender differences and changes in time use within urban and rural households in China

	2008			2017		
	Male	Female	Female/male	Male	Female	Female/male
Urban households						
Paid labor	5.45	4.06	0.74	7.24	4.95	0.68
Unpaid labor	1.91	4.24	2.22	1.28	3.64	2.84
#Housework	1.44	3.42	2.37	0.74	2.37	3.20
#Care for family members	0.42	0.75	1.79	0.54	1.27	2.35
Total labor	7.36	8.29	1.13	8.52	8.59	1.01
Leisure	4.90	4.04	0.83	4.18	3.84	0.92
Self-care	11.66	11.57	0.99	11.20	11.46	1.02
Labor force participation rate (%)	82.9	69.8	−13.1	86.9	67.1	−19.8
Monthly labor income (Yuan)	2226	1616	0.73	4349	3345	0.77
Observed value	6691	6691		1303	1303	
Rural households						
Paid labor	8.05	5.84	0.73	7.45	5.49	0.74
Unpaid labor	1.12	4.01	3.57	0.91	3.73	4.10
#Housework	0.83	3.37	4.07	0.69	2.71	3.93
#Care for family members	0.21	0.58	2.76	0.22	1.03	4.68
Total labor	9.17	9.84	1.07	8.36	9.22	1.10
Leisure	3.16	2.81	0.89	3.89	3.24	0.83
Self-care	11.63	11.31	0.97	11.65	11.42	0.98
Labor force participation rate (%)	95.3	89.4	−5.9	93.7	82.1	−11.6
Monthly labor income (Yuan)	959	645	0.67	2722	2140	0.79
Observed value	5816	5816		705	705	

Unit: hours/day
Source The 2008 and 2017 Chinese Time Use Surveys

women declined in rural areas, but also the labor force participation rate of males declined, only slightly less than that of females. In 2017, the labor force participation rate of rural residents remained significantly higher than that of urban residents, at 93.7% for rural males, 6.8% points higher than that of urban males, and 82.1% for rural females, 15% points higher than that of urban females. Similar to the urban situation, both men and women spent less time on unpaid labor (0.21 h per day for men and 0.28 h per day for women), but the ratio of women's to men's unpaid labor increased slightly, from 0.73 to 0.74. Unlike the urban population, where total labor time increased, the rural population experienced a decrease in total labor time, with men experiencing a greater decrease than women (0.81 h per day for men and 0.62 h per day for women). The ratio of women's to men's total labor time increased from 1.07 to 1.10. As total labor time became more unequally distributed, and leisure time became more unequally distributed between the sexes.

Comparing the data for urban and rural households in Table 5.3, we see that the urban–rural differences in labor force participation rate, paid labor time, unpaid labor time, and total labor time have significantly narrowed, and economic development has reduced the labor burden of rural residents, giving them more time to enjoy the leisure and care for their families (mainly children). However, the welfare enhancement of rural women was not as large as that of men, the total labor time of rural women was longer relative to that of men, and the gender difference in unpaid labor time has widened.

The Impact of Preschool Children on Gender Differences in Household Time Use

Childbearing is a factor that women must consider to balance work and family, and factors such as the presence or absence of minor children, the number of children, and the age of children can have an impact on household time allocation. Table 5.4 reports the effect of the presence or absence of children aged 0–6 years on intra-household time use.

As shown in Table 5.4, there is a more pronounced tendency for the gender division of labor to return to the traditional gender division of labor pattern in households with children aged 0–6 years. The male labor force participation rate in households with preschool-age children increased from 87.1% in 2008 to 91.2% in 2017, while the female labor force participation rate decreased from 73.0 to 66.1%, with the gender labor force participation rate difference reaching 25.1% points, which was 11% points higher than in 2008. In terms of time allocation, men's paid labor hours increased by 0.95 h per day and unpaid labor decreased by 0.40 h; women's paid labor hours decreased by 0.04 h per day and unpaid labor increased by 0.26 h. The result was that the gender ratio of paid labor hours decreased from 0.65 to 0.56, while the gender ratio of unpaid labor hours increased from 2.68 to 3.58. In terms of total labor hours, the total labor hours increased for both males and females, but the gender difference decreased, with the gender ratio of total labor hours decreasing from 1.11 to 1.07. The decrease in the gender difference in total labor hours was mainly due to the fact that the increase in paid labor hours for men exceeded the increase in unpaid labor time for women, and the gender difference in paid and unpaid labor time becomes larger.

The gender differences in time use for households without children aged 0–6 were similar to those for double-income households. Both men and women saw an increase in paid labor hours and a decrease in unpaid labor hours, with total labor

Table 5.4 Gender differences and changes in time use within Chinese families with and without children aged 0–6 years

Unit: hours/day

	2008			2017		
	Male	Female	Female/male	Male	Female	Female/male
With children of 0–6 years old						
Paid labor	6.44	4.19	0.65	7.39	4.15	0.56
Unpaid labor	1.89	5.07	2.68	1.49	5.33	3.58
#Housework	1.14	5.07	2.68	1.49	5.33	3.58
#Care for family members	0.68	1.66	2.54	0.92	3.05	3.32
Total labor	8.34	9.26	1.11	8.89	9.48	1.07
Leisure	3.86	3.11	0.81	3.34	2.65	0.79
Self-care	11.75	11.57	0.99	11.67	11.76	1.01
Labor force participation rate (%)	87.1	73.0	−14.1	91.2	66.1	−25.1
Monthly labor income (Yuan)	1582	1141	0.72	4627	4009	0.87
Observed value	3026	3026		446	446	
With no children of 0–6 years old						
Paid labor	6.72	5.11	0.76	7.32	5.53	0.76
Unpaid labor	1.43	3.83	2.67	0.99	3.18	3.21
#Housework	1.16	3.41	2.93	0.76	2.61	3.42
#Care for family members	0.21	0.35	1.67	0.23	0.57	2.48
Total labor	8.16	8.94	1.10	8.31	8.70	1.05
Leisure	4.16	3.57	0.86	4.26	3.84	0.90
Self-care	11.62	11.41	0.98	11.32	11.34	1.00
Labor force participation rate (%)	89.1	80.0	−8.3	89.6	76.7	−12.9
Monthly labor income (Yuan)	1662	1194	0.72	3739	2892	0.77
Observed value	9481	9481		1562	1562	

Source The 2008 and 2017 Chinese Time Use Surveys

hours increasing from 8.16 to 8.31 h per day for males and decreasing from 8.94 to 8.70 h per day for females due to different magnitudes of change. In relative terms, the ratio of paid labor time for women to men remained the same at 0.76, the ratio of unpaid labor time increased from 2.67 to 3.21, and the ratio of total labor time decreased from 1.10 to 1.05. Although total labor time was more evenly distributed between the sexes, women still worked 0.39 h more per day than men in absolute terms. Compared with households with children aged 0–6 years, couples without children aged 0–6 years have less total working time, with men working 0.58 h less per day and women working 0.78 h less per day; in other words, couples without children aged 0–6 years have more time to enjoy leisure.

Gender Differences in Time Use Within Households of Different Education Levels

This subsection compares gender differences and trends in time use within households of different education levels. The sample households were divided into three categories according to the husband's education levels: junior high school and below, high school and secondary vocational high school, and college and above. Table 5.5 reports the time use within these three categories of households.[15]

Table 5.5 shows that regardless of education level, time allocation within Chinese households has the following characteristics: women have shorter paid labor time, longer unpaid labor time, longer total labor time, and shorter leisure time compared to men. However, the gender differences in the division of labor generally tend to decrease as the education level increases. 2008 data show that in households with education levels of junior high school and below, high school and junior college, and college and above, the ratios of paid labor time for women and men were 0.70, 0.75, and 0.82, respectively, while the ratios of unpaid labor time were 3.11, 2.48, and 2.13, respectively, and the ratios of total labor time were 1.08, 1.12, and 1.14, respectively, which were opposite to the trend of gender differences in paid and unpaid labor time. In terms of the absolute amount of total labor time, women whose husbands had college or higher education worked 1.03 h more per day than their husbands, and women whose husbands had high school and junior college education worked 0.93 h more per day, and women whose husbands had a junior college education or less worked 0.67 h more per day. The reason for this phenomenon may be that as husbands' education levels increased, both husbands' paid labor time decreased, but husbands' paid labor time decreased more than wives', while unpaid labor time did not change much, resulting in the gender difference in total labor time widening with the increase of education level.

In 2017, among the three types of households with different education levels, both men and women saw an increase in paid labor hours and a decrease in unpaid labor hours, but the gender differences in time use changed significantly. The division of labor within households with a college degree and above has obviously returned to the traditional pattern. Compared with 2008, the labor participation rate of men increased from 90.8 to 95.8%, while that of women decreased from 81.4 to 78.6%, and the gender gap widened from 9.4 to 17.2% points; the ratio of paid labor time between women and men decreased from 0.82 to 0.73. The ratio of unpaid labor time increased from 2.13 to 2.59, and the ratio of total labor time decreased from 1.14 to

[15] If divided by the wife's education level, there would be fewer sample households with the education levels of college and above.

Table 5.5 Gender differences and changes in the time use of households by education level

Unit: hours/day

	2008			2017		
	Male	Female	Female/male	Male	Female	Female/male
Junior high school and below						
Paid labor	7.30	5.10	0.70	7.32	5.28	0.72
Unpaid labor	1.36	4.23	3.11	1.07	3.74	3.50
#Housework	1.03	3.54	3.44	0.72	2.61	3.63
#Care for family members	0.25	0.62	2.48	0.35	1.13	3.23
Total labor	8.66	9.33	1.08	8.39	9.02	1.08
Leisure	3.64	3.26	0.90	4.03	3.47	0.86
Self-care	11.67	11.37	0.97	11.48	11.40	0.99
Labor force participation rate (%)	88.7	79.4	−9.3	88.9	75.7	−13.2
Observed value	6478	6478		1248	1248	
High school and secondary vocational high school						
Paid labor	6.22	4.66	0.75	7.45	4.86	0.65
Unpaid labor	1.68	4.16	2.48	1.13	3.80	3.36
#Housework	1.31	3.44	2.63	0.77	2.63	3.42
#Care for family members	0.32	0.67	2.09	0.35	1.17	3.34
Total labor	7.90	8.83	1.12	8.58	8.66	1.01
Leisure	4.46	3.65	0.82	4.26	3.96	0.93
Self-care	11.56	11.45	0.99	11.06	11.27	1.02
Labor force participation rate (%)	86.8	76.0	−10.8	88.4	65.4	−23.0
Observed value	3358	3358		422	422	
College and above						
Paid labor	5.65	4.64	0.82	7.27	5.33	0.73
Unpaid labor	1.81	3.85	2.13	1.26	3.26	2.59
#Housework	1.27	3.00	2.13	1.26	3.26	2.59
#Care for family members	0.50	0.80	1.60	0.61	1.18	1.93
Total labor	7.46	8.49	1.14	8.53	8.59	1.01
Leisure	4.70	3.75	0.80	3.85	3.47	0.90
Self-care	11.71	11.63	0.99	11.51	11.83	1.03
Labor force participation rate (%)	90.8	81.4	−9.4	95.8	78.6	−17.2
Observed value	2671	2671		337	337	

Source The 2008 and 2017 Chinese Time Use Surveys

1.01; in terms of the absolute amount of total labor time, women worked on average 1.03 h more than men per day in 2008, while the total labor time of women was only 0.06 h more than men in 2017.

Similar to households with college and above, the labor force participation rate of men in households with high school and secondary vocational school increased, while the labor force participation rate of women decreased significantly (from 76.0 to 63.8%), and the gender gap widened from 10.8 to 23% points; the ratio of paid labor time of women to men decreased from 0.75 to 0.65, the ratio of unpaid labor time increased from 2.48 to 3.36, and the total labor time ratio fell from 1.12 to 1.01; in terms of the absolute amount of total labor time, women worked on average 0.93 h more than men per day in 2008, while the total labor time of women was only 0.08 h more than that of men in 2017.

Unlike the above two types of higher education households, in households with junior high school and below, although the female labor force participation rate also declined, the ratio of female to male paid labor time increased instead of declining, from 0.70 to 0.72. Like the other two types of households, the ratio of female to male unpaid labor time also increased from 3.10 to 3.50 in households with education levels junior high school and below. Although the total labor time of both males and females decreased, the relative contribution of women to the paid and unpaid labor of the household increased, and the total labor time of women was still 0.63 h per day more than that of men, and the ratio of total labor time to that of men remained unchanged at 1.08.

A comparison of families with different education levels reveals the dilemma faced by Chinese women: once society regards child and elderly care as "the private business of the family" and a "women's duty", even though the pursuit of gender equality in the labor market could help reduce women's economic dependence and improve their bargaining power, women were forced to bear the "double pressure" of work and family and did not have enough time to rest and enjoy leisure. While the pursuit of gender equality in the labor market could help reduce women's economic dependence and increase women's bargaining power, it left women with the "double burden" of work and family, without enough time to rest and enjoy leisure. For women in high-educated families, some of them can choose to "return to the family" due to their husbands' high income, which led to the waste of human capital; while for most women living in families with low or middle levels of education (low and middle income families) in China, they were still under the "double pressure" of work and family. While economic development has somehow reduced the total labor burden on women by reducing housework, it has not fundamentally changed the dilemma faced by Chinese women.

International Comparison of Gender Division of Labor

The distribution of labor time among residents across countries varies significantly due to the different perceptions of time use, the social division of labor, and gender inequality. In this section, these countries were selected: high welfare countries, such as Sweden; developed countries, such as the G7 countries (the United States, Canada, France, Germany, the United Kingdom, Japan, and Italy); transitional countries, such as Poland and Hungary; and East Asian countries which are geographically and culturally close to China, such as South Korea and Japan, as control groups to compare with the gender differences in time use of Chinese residents in 2008 and 2017. By comparing the gender differences in time use across countries, we can further understand the relationship between gender differences in time use and gender equality within households, see the gap with advanced countries, learn from the experiences of other countries, and promote gender equality in China.

Table 5.6 reports these countries' gender equality rankings, gender equality index, male and female labor force participation rates, female-to-male wage ratios, and fertility rates. Among these countries, Sweden, France, Germany, the United Kingdom, Canada, Poland, and the United States rank high in gender equality. These countries also have somewhat higher fertility rates than other countries except Germany and Poland. In contrast, Italy, Hungary, Japan, and South Korea rank low, and these countries also have lower fertility rates.

Next, the gender differences in paid and unpaid labor time in these countries are analyzed in relation to the degree of gender equality. Table 5.7 reports the average daily hours of paid and unpaid labor for men and women in the related countries. Data for countries other than China were obtained from a background paper written by Jacques Charmes for the 2015 UNDP Human Development Report Office.[16] The author received these data from the websites of statistics of the countries concerned, while the timing of the Time Use Survey and age groups of the respondents were not the same.[17] As micro data was not available, no corresponding adjustments were made in this paper. Although the different age groups of the sample affected the comparability of the data across countries to some extent, gender differences in time use between countries are still evident in the gender gap and ratio of labor hours. Given that most of the sample ages in the relevant countries in Table 5.7 were people aged 15 years and above, this section's sample ages were 15–74 years old from the 2008 and 2017 Chinese Time Use Survey. The 2017 sample included 29 provinces.

Table 5.7 shows that in all countries, women spent less time in paid labor than men, more time in unpaid labor than men, and more time in total labor than men.

[16] Jacques Charmes, "Time Use across the World: Findings of a World Compilation of Time Use Survey", UNDP Human Development Report Office Background Paper, 2015.

[17] Ages of the respondents selected for each country were as follows: Sweden 2010 (20–84 years old), USA 2014 (15 years old and above), Canada 2010 (15 years old and above), France 2010 (15 years old and above), Germany 2001–2002 (10 years old and above), UK 2005 (15 years old and above), Italy 2008–2009 (15 years old and above), Poland 2003–2004 (15–64 years old), Hungary 1999–2000 (15–74 years old), and Japan 2011 (10 years old and above), China 2008 (15–74 years old), China 2017 (15–74 years old), and Korea 2009 (10 years old and above).

Table 5.6 Gender equality indicators of relevant countries (2017)

Country	Global ranking	Gender equality index	Labor force participation rate (%)		Female/male wage ratio	Fertility rate
			Male	Female		
Sweden	5	0.816	84.1	79.8	0.74	1.91
France	11	0.778	75.1	67.2	0.47	1.98
Germany	12	0.778	82.6	73.1	0.68	1.46
The United Kingdom	15	0.770	82.6	71.9	0.67	1.87
Canada	16	0.769	81.5	74.4	0.68	1.58
Poland	39	0.728	75.5	62.0	0.55	1.30
The United States of America	49	0.718	77.4	66.2	0.73	1.87
Italy	82	0.692	73.7	54.3	0.49	1.47
China	100	0.674	84.3	70.3	0.64	1.62
Hungary	103	0.670	74.4	61.6	0.49	1.37
Japan	114	0.657	85.0	66.4	0.67	1.46
Republic of Korea	118	0.650	76.4	55.9	0.51	1.30

Source 2017 World Economic Forum: *The Global Gender Gap Report 2017*

Compared with other countries, Sweden, which ranked highest in gender equality, had the smallest gender differences in both types of labor time, with women spending 0. 66 h less per day in paid labor than men, 0.77 h more in unpaid labor than men, and 0.11 h more in total labor hours than men. Except for Italy and Japan, the other five G7 countries with high gender equality rankings had larger gender differences than Sweden, with women spending 1.25–1.47 h less per day in paid labor than men, 1.45–1.69 h more in unpaid labor, and 0.03–0.37 h more in overall labor time. Compared with the countries mentioned above, gender differences were larger in the two transitional countries: women in Poland and Hungary had 1.63 and 1.50 h less paid labor time per day than men, 2.30 and 2.35 h more unpaid labor time, and 0.67 and 0.85 h more of the total labor time, respectively. Among the G7 countries, Italy ranked lower in gender equality. It had a greater gender difference in the division of labor, with women working 2.00 h less per day in paid labor and 3.15 h more in unpaid labor than men; and women worked 1.15 h more per day than men in total labor hours. China's East Asian neighbors (Japan and Korea), which ranked lower than Italy in terms of gender equality, also had larger gender differences in the division of labor, with Japanese and Korean women working 2.75 and 1.68 h less per day in paid labor than men, and 2.95 and 2.48 h more per day in unpaid labor than men, respectively, while the gender differences in total labor time were relatively smaller in Japan than that in the Republic of Korea. Japanese women worked 0.20 h more than men per day, while Korean women worked 0.80 h more than men per

Table 5.7 Paid and unpaid labor time for women and men across countries

Unit: hours/day

	Male		Female	
	Paid labor	Unpaid labor	Paid labor	Unpaid labor
Sweden 2010	3.68	3.23	3.02	4.00
The United States of America 2014	4.28	2.65	2.93	4.10
Canada 2010	4.25	2.83	3.00	4.28
France 2010	3.32	2.47	2.10	3.90
Germany 2001–2002	3.70	2.28	2.23	3.78
The United Kingdom 2005	3.52	2.18	2.20	3.87
Italy 2008–2009	3.72	1.62	1.72	4.77
Poland 2003–2004	3.90	2.62	2.27	4.92
Hungary 1999–2000	4.35	2.12	2.85	4.47
Japan 2011	5.50	1.28	2.75	4.23
China 2017	6.03	1.13	4.19	3.37
China 2008	6.09	1.57	4.38	3.95
Republic of Korea 2009	4.10	0.65	2.42	3.13

Source Data for China are from the 2008 and 2017 Chinese Time Use Survey. Data for other countries are from Jacques Charmes, "Time Use across the World: Findings of a World Compilation of Time Use Survey", UNDP Human Development Report Office Background Paper, 2015

day. Compared with other countries, Korean men worked the least amount of unpaid labor time (0.65 h per day), followed by Chinese men in 2017 (1.13 h per day), and then followed by Japan and Italy of 1.28 h per day and 1.62 h per day, respectively.

Compared with the other countries in Table 5.7, the gender gap in labor time in China was similar to that in Poland and Hungary, the two transitional countries, and somewhat smaller than that in Italy, Japan, and Korea. Many transitional countries made great progress in gender equality in the labor market under the pre-transition socialist system. Still, they did not make corresponding progress in encouraging equal sharing of household work between men and women, so women faced the double burden of work and family. After the economic transition, the ideology of socialist gender equality faced great challenges, and the gender division of labor reverted to the traditional model of "men earn money to support the family while women take care of home".

Considering the different age groups of the Time Use Survey sample in different countries, countries whose samples included adolescents and the elderly would have somewhat fewer average labor hours than countries whose samples mainly covered the working age group. To reduce the effect of the absolute amount of time, Figs. 5.3, 5.4, and 5.5 report the ratio of paid labor time, the ratio of unpaid labor time, and the ratio of total labor time for females to males for each country, respectively. As can be seen from Fig. 5.3, the ratio of female to male paid labor time was less than 1 in all countries, but there were significant differences across countries, with four countries—Sweden, China, Canada, and the U.S.—having relatively small differences of the ratios of 0.82, 0.72 (decreasing to 0.69 in 2017), 0.71, and 0.68, respectively. The four countries with the largest differences were Italy, Japan, Poland, and the Republic of Korea, with ratios of 0.46, 0.50, 0.58, and 0.59, respectively.

From Fig. 5.4, we can see that in Sweden, Canada, and the United States, the gender differences were small in paid and unpaid labor, with female/male unpaid

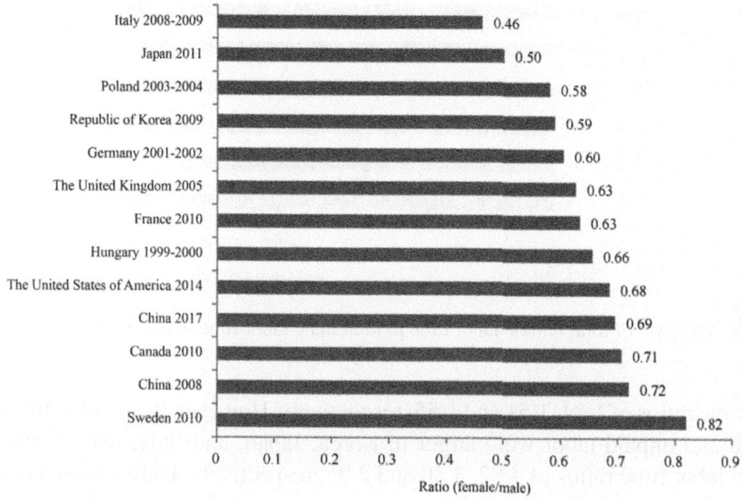

Fig. 5.3 The ratio of female paid labor time to male paid labor time in different countries

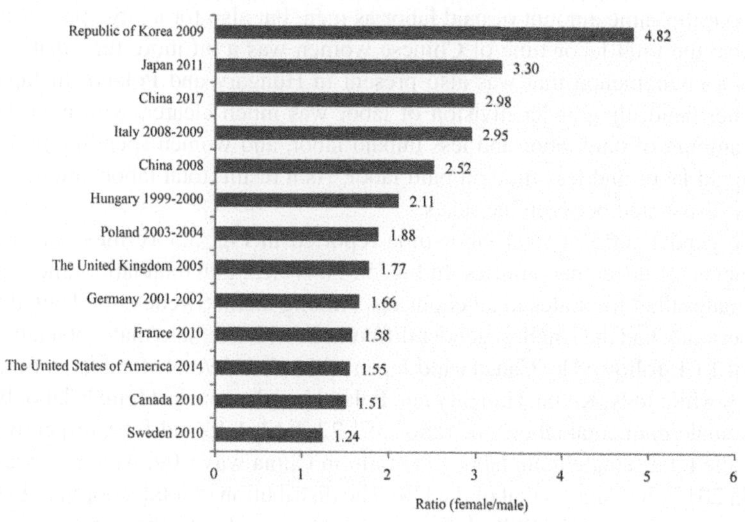

Fig. 5.4 The ratio of female unpaid labor time to male unpaid labor time in different countries

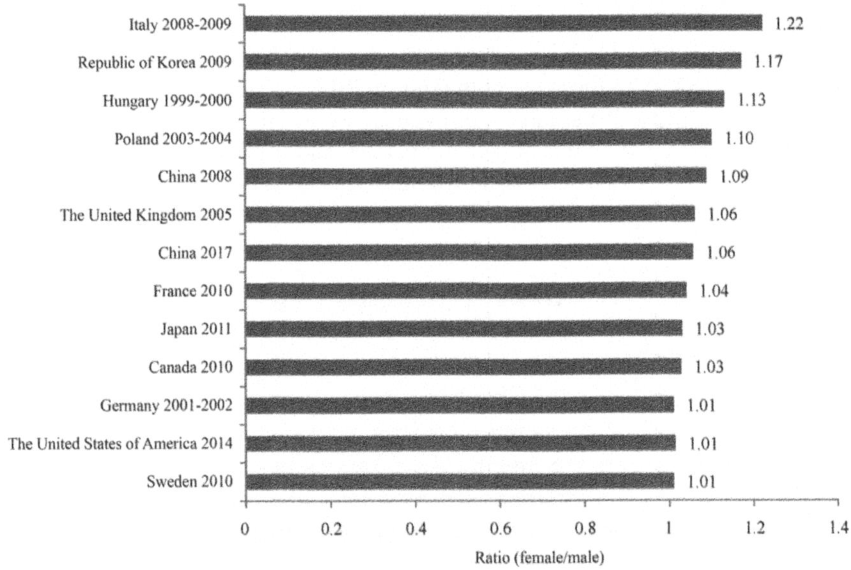

Fig. 5.5 The ratio of total female labor time to total male labor time in different countries

labor time ratios of 1.24, 1.51 and 1.55, respectively. However, the gender differences in paid and unpaid labor were larger in Korea, Japan, and Italy, with female/male unpaid labor time ratios of 4.82, 3.30 and 2.95, respectively. Unlike these countries, China had a smaller gender difference in paid labor, but a larger gender difference in unpaid labor, with the gender ratio of unpaid labor time being 2.52 in 2008 and rising to 2.98 in 2017, surpassing that of Italy. Chinese women were not only responsible for about the same amount of paid labor as men, but also for a large part of unpaid labor, so the total labor time of Chinese women was a bit more than that of men. It was a phenomenon that was also present in Hungary and Poland. In Japan, on the other hand, the gender division of labor was much clearer, with men doing a large amount of paid labor and less unpaid labor, and women spending more time on unpaid labor and less time on paid labor. As a result, total labor time was more evenly distributed between the sexes.

The gender ratio of total labor time reported in Fig. 5.5 verifies our previous judgments for different countries. In Fig. 5.5, it is clear that total labor time is higher for females than for males in all countries. Among them, Sweden, the United States and Germany had the smallest gender differences with a female/male total labor time ratio of 1.01, followed by Canada and Japan with a female/male total labor time ratio of 1.03, while Italy, Korea, Hungary and Poland had the heaviest female labor burden with female/male total labor time ratios of 1.22, 1.17, 1.13 and 1.10, respectively. In 2008, the total female/male labor time ratio in China was 1.09, which decreased to 1.06 in 2017, the same as that of the UK. The distribution of total labor time in China had become more even. Still, this evenness was not due to the narrowing gender differences in paid and unpaid labor time, but due to the widening gender differences in both types of labor time, and in this respect, the gender division of labor pattern within Chinese households was more similar to that of Japanese households.

Summary

This chapter analyzes and compares the changes in the time use of married men and women in China in 2008 and 2017. The analysis finds significant gender differences in the time use within Chinese households: compared with men, women spend far less time on paid labor, far more time on unpaid labor, slightly more time on total labor, and less time on leisure. Over the nine years from 2008 to 2017, the gender division of labor within Chinese households changed significantly. In general, the female/male ratio of paid labor time has become lower, the ratio of unpaid labor time has become higher, and the ratio of total labor time has decreased. These changes indicate that the division of labor within Chinese households tends to return to the traditional model that "men's work centers around outside, while women's work centers on home". In contrast, the distribution of total household labor time between the two sexes has become more even due to the withdrawal of some women of childbearing age from the labor market and the increase in income levels, which has reduced women's time spent on household chores. The "double burden" of work and family faced by Chinese women has been reduced.

However, changes in the gender division of labor within households varied greatly by social group, with the tendency to return to the traditional pattern of gender division of labor more pronounced in urban households than in rural households; more pronounced in households with preschool-age children than in households without preschool-age children, and more pronounced in households with senior high school or higher education levels than in households with junior high school or lower education levels. The return to the traditional gender division of labor reduced the total labor burden of females in urban and high-education households to some extent. In contrast, the female/male ratio of paid labor time increased for women in rural and low-education level households. At the same time, the female/male ratio of unpaid labor time also increased significantly, thus making their total labor burden heavier and the inequitable distribution of total labor time unimproved. For households with preschool-age children, the decrease in female labor force participation rate did not change the inequitable distribution of total labor time within the household, and the total labor time of females remained longer than that of males. A comparison of different types of households reveals the dilemma faced by married women in China: returning to the traditional family model reduces women's labor burden but increases their economic dependence; participating in the labor market to the same extent as men helps increase women's economic empowerment, but they have to endure the "double burden" of work and family, lacking sufficient leisure time.

Comparisons with G7 and transitional countries show that countries with high gender equality also have smaller gender differences in labor time, not only in terms of gender differences in paid and unpaid labor time, but also in terms of the more equal distribution of total labor time between the sexes. Countries with low gender equality have larger gender differences in labor time. Japan has more symmetrical gender differences between the two types of labor and therefore smaller gender differences in total labor time, while Italy, Korea, Poland and Hungary have asymmetrical gender differences between paid and unpaid labor, with the result that the gender differences in total labor time are larger. In 2008, China's gender division of labor within households was similar to Poland and Hungary, the two transitional countries. Going into 2017, the gender division of labor within Chinese households was similar to the Japanese household pattern.

The changing trend of gender division of labor within Chinese households should be of great concern to policymakers. The withdrawal of women from the labor market and their return to the family run counter to the general trend of the international community to promote gender equality and will have a negative impact on China's achievement of the UN 2030 Sustainable Development Goals. In the face of China's aging population, the net demand for female labor in the labor market has increased (as evidenced by a narrowing gender wage gap), while the return of women to the family will exacerbate labor shortages and reduce the rate of economic growth. In addition, facing the double burden of work and family, some women from high-income households can choose to return to their families, but it is difficult for women from low-income households to make this choice; their withdrawal from the labor market will exacerbate the economic stratification of Chinese families, but if they stay in the labor market, they will face a heavy labor burden with no spare time to enhance their labor productivity. Finally, the experience of developed countries tells us that the dilemma of married women will greatly reduce young women's willingness to marry and have children, which will further reduce China's fertility rate.

Experience in developed countries shows that reducing gender disparities in work hours within families requires the state to guarantee equal employment rights for women with family responsibilities. Public investment in childcare institutions and preschool education should be increased, maternity insurance coverage should be improved, "family-friendly" labor arrangements should be promoted, and men should be encouraged to share more of the domestic and family care responsibilities. The changes in China's household time use in this chapter also suggest that economic development, improved living standards, and the marketization of household services have also helped to reduce married women's housework, alleviating the "double burden" they face at work and at home and allowing them to have more leisure time.

Part III
Winning at the Starting Line: Education and Development in China

Chapter 6
Equity in Educational from the Perspective of the Time Use of School-Age Children

Education directly affects people's income and welfare, and equity in education is an important part of achieving social justice. Education is a long-term process of accumulating human capital for each person in the early and middle stages of the life cycle. The education level at each stage is a prerequisite for entering the next stage of education. The existence of externalities also makes the benefits generated by the investment in education at each stage incremental in nature. The difference in educational investments directly leads to inequity at the start of education, which also causes the continuous expansion of the human capital gap in subsequent stages and eventually leads to social inequality. Hence, it is especially important to study the impact of the difference in starting point on education inequity.

Investments in education can be divided into public and household investments. Public investment in education can compensate for the lack of family investment to a certain extent. China has taken several policy measures to provide every child with a fair opportunity for education and improve the nation's overall education level. Chapter five of the *Common Program of the Chinese People's Political Consultative Conference*, promulgated in 1949, clearly stipulates that "compulsory education shall be made universal in a planned and systematic manner" throughout the country. At the National People's Congress held in April 1986, the Compulsory Education Law of the People's Republic of China was passed, universalizing education at the primary and junior high school levels nationwide; the main goal of the *Opinions on the Implementation of the Third Phase of Preschool Education* promulgated by the Ministry of Education in 2017 is "to basically build a public service system of preschool education with wide coverage, basic protection and quality by 2020. By that means, the national preschool's three-year net enrollment rate should reach 85%, the coverage rate of inclusive kindergartens should reach about 80%, the basic quality of kindergarten teachers should be improved, the basic form of the kindergarten quality assessment and supervision system should be built, and the general standardization of school behavior should be implemented." In 2017, the Ministry of Education promulgated the *Guideline for Popularizing High School Education (2017–2020)* to achieve nationwide education of senior high schools by 2020. The

F. Du et al., *Chinese People's Time Use and Their Quality of Life*,
https://doi.org/10.1007/978-981-99-5526-8_6

United Nations *2030 Agenda for Sustainable Development* lists "ensuring inclusive and equitable quality education and lifelong learning opportunities for all" as one of the 17 Sustainable Development Goals (SDGs); target 4.1 of which is to "ensure that all children complete primary and secondary education that is free, equitable and of good quality, with relevant and effective learning outcomes by 2030"; target 4.2 calls for ensuring that all children have access to quality early childhood development, care and preschool education to prepare them for primary education.

The United Nations General Assembly adopted the *Convention on the Rights of the Child* on November 20, 1989, defining a child as any person under the age of 18. Based on the UN *Convention on the Rights of the Child* and the reality that Chinese children complete high school education at the age of roughly 18, we define children as residents aged 18 and under. Using data from the 2017 Chinese Time Use Survey, this chapter uses a sample of school-age children aged 3–18 to examine the learning time of children in China from preschool to senior high school. It also examines the current state of education equity in China from three perspectives: urban and rural areas, mothers' education levels, and household income levels. Here, we divide learning activities into three stages: classroom, homework, and extracurricular tutoring. Among them, classroom activities include two types: attending classes at school and extracurricular activities organized by schools. Specifically, classroom activities include: attending classes and lectures at school, taking exams, having breaks, doing exercises, and class-related waiting and transportation activities. Extracurricular activities include gardening and tree-planting, sports, cultural, and public welfare activities. Homework activities include: reading literature, writing papers, doing experiments and other research activities; completing after-school homework; reviewing and pre-reading homework and related transportation activities. Extracurricular tutoring, also known as "shadow education", refers to the paid educational activities conducted outside of school education. In the 2017 Chinese Time Use Survey data, extracurricular tutoring activities include: taking classes and tutors; classes and tutors for the purpose of art and sports examinations; and other audio, physical and aesthetic classes and tutors and related transportation activities. These three types of activities require investment from both the school and the family, but the two sides play different roles in each category. For example, while classes and homework are arranged by schools and teachers and also require parental supervision and individual child effort, extracurricular tutoring relies heavily on parental financial investment and child participation, which is particularly important for kindergarten and elementary school students. After-school tutoring services are far more available in urban than in rural areas; highly educated mothers and high-income families are better equipped to send their children to after-school tutoring to supervise and help them with their homework than low-educated mothers and low-income families. In summary, a family's socioeconomic status affects the amount of time children spend studying and leads to the intergenerational transmission of education inequality.

Basic Information on School-Age Children's Time Use

In China, the 3–18 age group covers roughly all school-age children from kindergarten to senior high school, and we divide children's ages into 3–6 preschool stage, 7–12 elementary school stage, 13–15 junior high school age, and 16–18 senior high school age. In the 2017 Chinese Time Use Survey data, we selected children whose status was a student (3–18 years old) and for which parental and family information could be tracked, totaling a sample of 3854 children. Since we mainly discuss education equity by analyzing the study time of the school-age population, the number of people covered in this chapter does not include students who were on vacation. Divided by residence and gender, the sample in this chapter contains 1,457 rural and 2,397 urban students, among which 2,055 were boys, and 1,799 were girls. Mothers' education levels were divided into four categories: elementary school and below, junior high school, senior high school/junior college, and college and above. The sample households were divided into three categories based on quintiles of household per capita income distribution in each province: the lowest 20%, the middle 60%, and the highest 20%.

Table 6.1 reports the time use of children aged 3–18 years in China from perspectives of gender, urban and rural areas, mothers' education level, and household income. During the 24-h day, children's activities are divided into four categories: self-care, learning, playing, and others. Self-care is the activity that all people must do to meet their basic needs for survival, including sleeping, eating, and personal hygiene activities. Learning is the primary daily activity of school-age children and is examined in detail in this chapter, including classes, extracurricular tutoring, and homework activities. Playing mainly includes all forms of recreational and leisure activities, sports and fitness activities, reading unrelated to schoolwork and further studies, and non-school organized sports and fitness activities. Other activities include all activities other than those mentioned above, such as housework, caring for family members and shopping.

For school-age children, studying is the most important activity each day, spending an average of 7.30 h, or 63.1% of all time in the day, except for self-care activities. Among these, 62.4 and 63.8% of a whole day time were spent by boys and girls, respectively, which shows that girls studied more than boys, and were higher than boys in terms of length and percentage of time spent on study. However, the school-age children's study time by gender was not significant. There was a big difference between urban and rural areas in terms of the participation length of study and percentage of time spent, with rural children studying 6.93 h, 0.61 h less than urban children, and 5.2% less than urban children. In Section Three, we will discuss the differences in learning activities between rural and urban school-age children.

As mothers' education level increased, children's learning hours were 7.17, 7.29, 7.41 and 7.37 h, and the percentages of learning hours spent were 61.1, 63.1, 64.3 and 65.2%. Therefore, the percentage of children's learning hours was greater in families with better-educated mothers and less in families with mothers of low education levels, with a significant intergenerational transmission of educational activities.

Table 6.1 Average participation length of main activities for school-age children. Unit: hours/day

	Self-care	Studying	Playing	Others	Total time
The whole country	12.44	7.30	3.67	0.59	24
Boys	12.34	7.27	3.83	0.57	24
Girls	12.55	7.30	3.54	0.61	24
Rural	12.45	6.93	3.98	0.64	24
Urban	12.43	7.54	3.47	0.56	24
Average participation length of primary activity for school-age children by mother's education levels					
Primary school and below	12.27	7.17	3.75	0.81	24
Junior high school	12.44	7.29	3.73	0.54	24
Senior high school/junior college	12.48	7.41	3.65	0.46	24
College and above	12.69	7.37	3.46	0.48	24
Average participation length of primary activity for school-age children by income levels					
The lowest 20%	12.24	7.06	3.94	0.58	24
The middle 60%	12.45	7.31	3.65	0.59	24
The highest 20%	12.41	7.50	3.47	0.62	24

The impact of household income per capita on children's study time was more obvious. As household income increased, children's study hours were 7.06, 7.31 and 7.50 h, and the percentages of children's study time were 61.0, 63. 3 and 64.7%, with a stepwise increase. Children in higher-income families spent more time studying and a higher percentage of study hours.

Table 6.2 reports the average participation length and rates of learning activities for school-age children. As can be seen, learning activities were dominated by public education such as attending classes at school and supplemented by private education such as extracurricular tutoring, with classes accounting for 80.3% of total learning hours and extracurricular tutoring accounting for 3%. The national average length of school-age children's lessons was 5.86 h, with a participation rate of 71.4%, while extracurricular tutoring time was 0.22 h and homework time was 1.22 h. Boys had a higher average length and participation rate in class than girls, while girls had a higher average length and participation rate in total learning, extracurricular tutoring, and homework activities than boys. Analysis of learning activities at different age levels revealed that the amount of time spent in class increased with age, and the relationship between attending class and doing homework was synchronous; the longer the time spent in class, the longer the time spent doing homework.

In terms of educational stages, the number of hours spent on learning at the primary, junior high and senior high school levels were 7.30 h, 8.78 h and 8. 80 h, respectively. It can be seen that senior high school students spent the longest time studying, followed by junior high school students and elementary school students. Overall, elementary school students spent the longest time attending extracurricular tutoring and junior high school students spent the longest time doing homework.

Table 6.2 Average length and participation rates of learning activities for school-age children

	Average hours per day				Participation rate (%)		
	Taking classes	Extracurricular tutoring	Doing homework	Total	Taking classes	Extracurricular tutoring	Doing homework
The whole country	5.86	0.22	1.22	7.30	71.4	6.0	53.8
Boys	5.96	0.19	1.12	7.27	73.1	5.5	21.6
Girls	5.73	0.24	1.33	7.30	69.4	6.6	56.4
3–6 years old	4.81	0.08	0.24	5.13	68.0	2.2	19.4
7–12 years old	5.53	0.32	1.45	7.30	72.9	9.4	70.0
13–15 years old	6.74	0.28	1.76	8.78	73.1	6.7	66.8
16–18 years old	7.19	0.11	1.50	8.80	71.0	2.7	52.0

Time spent in school was consistently the longest in all three stages of learning activities, accounting for 75.6, 76.8, and 81.7%. The difference is that the length of time spent in class and doing homework was shorter in elementary school than in junior high school and senior high school, but longer in extracurricular tutoring than those two, with an average of 0.32 h, 1.14 times than that of junior high school and 3 times that of the senior high school. On August 22nd, 2013, the Ministry of Education issued the *Ten Rules for Reducing the Burden of Elementary School Students* to reduce the excessive burden of schoolwork on elementary school students in terms of homework, exams and work and rest, but the data showed that "reducing the burden" has not been achieved in a real sense. "There is no homework in school, so naturally, students will search elsewhere to make up." Participating in extracurricular tutoring courses has become the choice of many parents. Students' learning pressure did not reduce. At the same time, parents' economic burden has increased a lot. The phenomenon of "the school reduces the burden, while the community increases the burden" and "teachers reduce the burden, while parents increase the burden" have already appeared.

Rural Areas Fail to Keep up with Urban Areas in Achieving Equity at the Starting Point of Children's Educational Development

This section focuses on the learning situation of school-age children living in towns and rural areas. Compulsory education is a mandatory national education for school-age children and must be guaranteed by the state, society, schools, and families.

Table 6.3 Net enrollment rate of school-age children. Unit: %

	National total	Urban	Rural
3–6 years old	71.3	76.4	63.1
7–12 years old	97.5	98.0	96.9
13–15 years old	97.0	97.4	96.4
16–18 years old	91.1	91.3	90.8

It is the state's most robust measure to ensure schooling opportunities for school-age children by law. The government's legal responsibility is to provide primary and balanced compulsory education. Every school-age child should enjoy equal opportunity to receive mandatory education of quality. Its nature determines that compulsory education must be developed in a balanced manner.

The difference in government policies and investments is one of the critical factors affecting equity in education for school-age children. Compared with non-compulsory education, the state's public investment is presented through national policies, investment in education, building schools, and staffing of teachers. Many studies at home and abroad have shown that government investment in education is one of the main reasons affecting children's future education level and income. Increasing enrollment is also an effective measure to promote educational equity and narrow the gap between urban and rural education.[1]

Table 6.3 reports the net enrollment rate of school-age children. Regarding school-age enrollment, the compulsory education stage had the highest net enrollment rate, with the 7–12 and 13–15 years old groups having the highest net enrollment rates. The net enrollment rates for students aged 7–12 and 13–15 were above 97%, indicating that the effect of compulsory education in China was relatively significant. In the non compulsory education stage, the net enrollment rate of preschool education was much lower than that of the compulsory education period, at 71.3%, with the net enrollment rate in urban areas at 76.4%, which was 13.3% points lower than that of 63.1% in urban areas. The net enrollment rate at the high school level dropped to 91.1%. The net enrollment rate of children showed an urban–rural disparity in children's education in China, with a more considerable disparity at the preschool level.

The preschool stage is the benchmark for influencing school enrollment and the most critical stage for developing various knowledge competencies and reducing differences in future human capital accumulation. The disparity between urban and rural preschool net enrollment rates reflects the fact that children's access to an equal education is very limited without the protection of compulsory education, and more rural children do not have access to good education. For this reason, many scholars have suggested that the preschool stage should be included in compulsory education. The other non-compulsory stage (senior high school level) has a significantly higher net enrollment rate than 3–6-year-olds due to the fact that the inclusion of

[1] Jun Yang, Xiao Huang, Xin Liu, "An Analysis of Education Inequality in China", *International Journal of Educational Development*, 2014, 37 (4).

senior high school in the compulsory education category has been an important issue since the universalization of compulsory education and has been piloted in some provinces, such as Hebei, Guangdong and some cities in the Inner Mongolia Autonomous Region. This action and trend have reduced the urban–rural enrollment gap accordingly. The Ministry of Education's plans for the twelve-year compulsory education, the *Plan of Solving Difficulties on the Popularization of Senior Secondary Education (2017–2020)*, will universalize senior high school education nationwide in 2020, with the focus on the poor areas in central and western China, ethnic areas, remote areas, old revolutionary areas, other areas with a weak foundation and low penetration of education, and concentrated contiguous areas with special difficulties. The focus is on special groups such as students from economically disadvantaged families, students with disabilities, and children of migrant workers in urban areas, etc. The key is to solve outstanding problems such as the high proportion of large classes in ordinary senior high schools, the continuous decline in the proportion of vocational education enrollment, and the difficulties in school operation.

Table 6.4 reports the average length of learning activities and participation rates for school-age children. The results for children divided by age stage in the text differ less from those obtained by education stages, so this chapter only presents the results by children's age. It can be seen that the difference between urban and rural children's total learning hours is significant, with urban children having more learning activities than rural children, with the largest difference at the age of 16–18 years, when urban children's total learning hours were 9.38 h, 1.39 h higher than that in rural areas. There was a polarization between compulsory and non-compulsory education, with rural children spending more time and participating in classes than urban children in compulsory education, and vice versa in non-compulsory education, especially in the 3–6-year-old stage, where rural children's participation rate was 62.2%, lower than that of the urban children by 9.2% points. This was related to the low net enrollment rate in rural kindergartens. Overall, the small gap between urban and rural children's school hours suggests that China's compulsory education policy ensures the right to education for all children and promotes education equity.

In terms of extracurricular tutoring time, urban and rural children had uneven opportunities. The average length and participation rate of urban children in extracurricular tutoring were higher than those of rural children in all age groups, and the proportion and length of participation of rural children in extracurricular tutoring were the highest in the 7–12 age group, but only a half of that of the urban children. The objective conditions for rural children to participate in extracurricular tutoring were insufficient. Most of the extracurricular tutoring institutions and teachers were concentrated in urban areas with higher levels of economic development, compared to rural areas where education levels were backward and extracurricular tutoring institutions and teachers were scarce. At the same time, the cost of extracurricular tutoring was very high, and the poor economic development of rural areas also

Table 6.4 Average participation length of learning activities and participation rate of school-age children

	Average hours per day				Participation rate (%)		
	Taking classes	Extracurricular tutoring	Doing homework	Total	Taking classes	Extracurricular tutoring	Doing homework
3–6 years old							
Rural	4.40	0.03	0.22	4.65	62.2	0.7	16.0
Urban	5.05	0.10	0.26	5.42	71.4	3.0	21.3
7–12 years old							
Rural	5.79	0.22	1.12	7.13	73.3	6.9	64.8
Urban	5.33	0.40	1.71	7.44	72.7	11.4	74.0
13–15 years old							
Rural	6.82	0.03	1.43	8.28	74.9	1.3	60.6
Urban	6.68	0.44	1.98	9.10	71.9	10.2	70.9
16–18 years old							
Rural	6.94	0.00	1.04	7.99	69.7	0.1	42.1
Urban	7.37	0.18	1.82	9.38	71.8	4.6	59.2

limited families' ability to pay for children's education.[2] The average time spent doing homework and extracurricular tutoring was similar, and the average length and participation rate of urban children doing homework was higher than that of rural children in all age groups, with the largest gap in the 16–18 age group, where the participation rate of urban children doing homework was 59.2%, 17.1% points higher than that of rural children.

Usually, the school-age population goes to classes. When the household income gap is large, public education plays a greater role in reducing education inequity than private education, such as extracurricular tutoring.[3] The implementation of legal policies and increased investment in public education has reduced urban–rural differences in compulsory school-age attendance, even to the extent that rural areas are slightly more likely than urban areas to attend classes in terms of hours and participation rates. In the non-compulsory education stage, where public investment is relatively low, urban areas are higher than rural areas in participation length and rates, with significant urban–rural differences. Therefore, increasing public investment in non-compulsory education plays a crucial role in improving educational equity, and this view is also consistent with the findings of domestic scholars.[4]

[2] Changgen Pei, Naiqing Song, Qiaohui Liu, "Empirical Analysis and Implications of Students' Participation in Extracurricular Tutoring at the Compulsory Education Stage," *Journal of The Chinese Society of Education*, 2018 (3).

[3] Gerhard Glomm, B. Ravikumar, "Public versus Private Investment in Human Capital: Endogenous Growth and Income Inequality", *Journal of Political Economy*, 1992, 100 (4).

[4] Kaimng Guo, Quanseng Zhang, Liutang Gong, "Public Policy, Economic Growth, and the Evolution of Inequality", *Economic Research Journal*, 2011, S2.

The Mother's Education Level Affects the Child's Educational Development

In family investments, parents' education level is an important factor that influences children's learning. Parents' education levels or parents' intellectual capital affects the learning achievement and future development of children in the family.[5] Intergenerational relationships in education also suggest that increasing parents' education level is an important means of improving educational equity, so the effect of equitable education has a sustained effect.[6] It has also been found that better educated mothers maintain communication with school teachers and focus more on children's advancement and various learning activities.[7]

Table 6.5 reports the net enrollment rates of school-age children by mother's education levels. As can be seen, there are significant differences in the net enrollment rates of children with different education levels from their mothers. For children aged 3–6, the higher the mother's education level, the higher the child's net enrollment rate. The net enrollment rate of children was 65.1% when the mother's education level was elementary school or below, with respective differences of 7.4, 11.0, and 12.2% points of net enrollment rates compared with the other three groups where the mother's education level was higher. It can be learned that the mother's low education severely affected the net enrollment rate of children aged 3–6. At the compulsory education level for ages 7–12 and 13–15, the mother's education level had little difference in the impact on children's net enrollment rate up to 95.7–98.8% in general. This shows that the implementation of compulsory education has reduced the impact of mothers' education level on children's net enrollment rates. The lowest net enrollment rate for children aged 16–18 was 87.2% when the mother's education level was elementary school or below. The difference between the net enrollment rate of children in the three groups with higher maternal education was 6.0, 7.2, and 5.3% points, respectively. Compared with children aged 3–6, the net enrollment rate for children aged 16–18 years varied between mothers' education. The difference is smaller, indicating that the mother's education level has a greater impact on preschool children's enrollment during the non-compulsory education period.

Table 6.6 reports the school-age children's learning by mothers' education level. All age groups show that the average participation length and rates of studying increased as the mother's education level increased. Especially for children aged 13–15, whose mothers' education level was college and above, the average participation length of study was 10.97 h, about 2.89 h higher than that of children whose mothers had primary education or below. The average participation length of study for 16–18 years old children whose mothers had college education or higher was 10.34 h,

---

[5] Annette Lareau, "Social Class Differences in Family-school Relationships: The Importance of Cultural Capital", *Sociology of Education*, 1987, 60 (4).

[6] Yunsen Li, Hao Qi, "Intergenerational Causality in Rural Education in China—A Study Based on the Universal Rural Basic Education Policy in the 1970s", *World Economic Papers*, 2011 (4).

[7] David P. Baker, David L. Stevenson, "Mother's Strategies for Children's School Achievement: Managing the Transition to High School", *Sociology of Education*, 1986, 59 (3).

Table 6.5 Net enrollment rates of school-age children by mother's education level. Unit: %

Age of children	Education level			
	Primary school and below	Junior high school	Senior high school/junior college	College and above
3–6 years old	65.1	72.5	76.1	77.3
7–12 years old	97.1	98.8	96.5	97.1
13–15 years old	95.7	98.3	98.5	96.7
16–18 years old	87.2	93.2	94.4	92.5

about 1.97 h higher than for children whose mothers had primary education or below. Most children in the 16–18 age group were enrolled in senior high school, which was a critical age for children to enter college through preparation for the college entrance exams. Children in this age group also spent the longest time in school as their mothers were better educated and focused on the children's further education and success. This is consistent with economic research findings.[8]

Extracurricular tutoring is an alternative way of studying besides going to school. In Table 6.6, we find that children's time spent in extracurricular tutoring increased as the mother's education level increased. When the mother's education level was college and above, the highest participation rate of children in extracurricular tutoring was 15. 1% at the age of 13–15, with an average participation length of 1.02 h, approximately 13 times the time spent by children whose mothers' education level was elementary school and below, 5 times the time spent by children whose mothers' education level was junior high school, and 3 times the time spent by children whose mothers' education level was senior high school. This suggests that parents with high levels of education compensate children the most outside of schooling. When the mother's education level was elementary school and below, children of all ages had significantly fewer hours of extracurricular tutoring and participation rates than other families with high educational backgrounds. Maybe this was because a low education level was usually associated with low household income, so the cost of extracurricular tutoring could not be afforded. Another reason was that parents in families with low educational backgrounds did not emphasize their children's education enough. Increased investment in public education can increase educational improvement and reduce the need for extracurricular tutoring fundamentally, while compensating for the pressure of low educational backgrounds on children's extracurricular tutoring, narrowing the educational gap between children from various family educational backgrounds, and reducing educational inequities.

Meanwhile, the participation length and rate of homework were more significantly influenced by mothers' education level, especially after age 7, when children's homework time increased more substantially as mothers' education level increased. At the age of 7–12, children whose mothers' education level was college and above

[8] C. Guitérrez, R. Tanakam, "Inequality and Education Decisions in Developing Countries", *Journal of Economic Inequality*, 2009, 7 (11).

Table 6.6 School-age children's learning by mother's education level

	Average hours per day				Participation rate (%)		
Education level	Taking classes	Extracurricular tutoring	Doing homework	Total	Taking classes	Extracurricular tutoring	Doing homework
3–6 years old							
Primary school and below	4.44	0.04	0.20	4.68	65.4	0.5	17.7
Junior high school	4.83	0.04	0.29	5.16	69.3	1.7	19.6
Senior high school/junior college	5.48	0.01	0.27	5.76	70.8	0.9	21.7
College and above	4.52	0.23	0.19	4.94	65.9	5.1	18.3
7–12 years old							
Primary school and below	5.74	0.09	1.17	7.00	73.2	2.9	62.7
Junior high school	5.56	0.33	1.46	7.35	73.0	9.8	71.0
Senior high school/junior college	5.47	0.36	1.47	7.30	75.4	11.7	70.8
College and above	5.01	0.80	2.03	7.84	69.1	20.7	82.4
13–15 years old							
Primary school and below	6.35	0.08	1.47	8.08	73.2	2.4	67.1
Junior high school	6.93	0.22	1.71	8.86	73.3	5.1	64.2
Senior high school/junior college	6.32	0.37	1.94	8.63	69.5	14.4	63.8
College and above	7.29	1.02	2.66	10.97	77.5	15.1	80.4

(continued)

Table 6.6 (continued)

	Average hours per day				Participation rate (%)		
Education level	Taking classes	Extracurricular tutoring	Doing homework	Total	Taking classes	Extracurricular tutoring	Doing homework
16–18 years old							
Primary school and below	7.10	0.01	1.26	8.37	72.4	0.1	44.6
Junior high school	6.83	0.22	1.38	8.43	67.7	5.2	51.6
Senior high school/ junior college	7.99	0.12	1.60	9.71	74.4	4.1	56.0
College and above	7.74	0.03	2.57	10.34	72.8	1.1	72.4

had 0.86 h more homework time than children whose mothers' education level was elementary school and below, with a 19.7% point higher participation rate. The largest average time difference between 13 and 15 years old was 1.19 h; the average time difference between 16 and 18 years old was 1.31 h. The participation rate of children doing homework in highly educated families was about 1.6 times higher than that in low-educated families. The higher the education level, the more parents perceive the return on investment in their children's education and are stricter with their children's learning requirements.

Family Income Differences Exacerbate Inequitable Opportunities for the Educational Development of School-Age Children

Education is an activity that entails significant human and financial costs. Some of these investments can be borne by the state and public bodies, and some by families. Among the costs that families invest are the time commitment of tutoring or caring for children and the financial costs of educating children. While higher-income families are more likely to provide better learning conditions and material resources for their children, children from low-income families lack access to quality education, face more family pressure, and have relatively less access to educational resources and educational experiences that can provide the motivational basis for children's

Table 6.7 Net enrollment of school-age children by income level. Unit: %

Age of children	Income		
	The lowest 20%	The middle 60%	The highest 20%
3–6 years old	62.1	72.8	78.7
7–12 years old	95.9	97.8	98.7
13–15 years old	96.5	97.1	97.3
16–18 years old	89.2	90.3	96.7

further learning later in life.[9] Therefore, children from high-income families are more invested in learning compared to children from low-income families.

Table 6.7 reports the net enrollment rates of school-age children by income level. As income increased, net enrollment rates for children of all ages increased significantly. Among the four age groups, the smaller disparities in net enrollment rates for children from different income households were found in the 7–12 and 13–15 years of compulsory education. The gap in net enrollment rates between high and low income families was within 2.8% points. The larger gaps were in the 3–6 and 16–18 years' group, which did not fall into the compulsory education category. The most notable difference between the net enrollment rates of high and low-income families was 16.6% points at the 36-year-old preschool level. The difference in net enrollment rates between high and low-income families at the high school level, ages 16–18, was 7.5%. Although smaller than the difference for children in the 3–6 years of age, the difference was smaller than that for children in the 3–6 years' age group, but the income level still affected their net enrollment rate relative to children in the compulsory education stage. This shows that children from low-income families who lacked public policy guarantees still had an inequitable chance to go to school.

Table 6.8 reports on school-age children's learning by income level. For children aged 3–6 years, income differences did not have a significant effect on the amount of time children spent in class. For children aged 7–12, the average length of time and participation in extracurricular tutoring and homework increased as household income increased, with children in high-income households attending extracurricular tutoring for 4.1 times longer than children in low-income households and children in middle-income families participated in extracurricular tutoring 2.3 times more than children in low-income families. Doing homework had the largest disparity across income families, with children in high-income families spending about 0.7 h more than those in low-income families. For 13–15-year-olds and 16–18-year-olds, the average length of time spent in class and doing homework and participation rates increased as household income increased.

[9] Leishan Shi, Yingmin Chen, Xiu Hou, Qiang Feng, "The Relationship Between Family Socioeconomic Status and Learning Engagement: The Mediating Role of Academic Self-Efficacy", *Psychological Development and Education*, 2013 (1).

Table 6.8 School-age children's learning by income level

Income	Average hours per day				Participation rate (%)		
	Taking classes	Extracurricular tutoring	Doing homework	Total	Taking classes	Extracurricular tutoring	Doing homework
3–6 years old							
The lowest 20%	4.83	0.10	0.27	5.20	68.0	3.3	20.1
The middle 60%	4.84	0.09	0.23	5.16	68.5	2.2	20.9
The highest 20%	4.71	0.03	0.27	5.01	66.3	1.0	12.7
7–12 years old							
The lowest 20%	5.85	0.14	1.24	7.23	74.8	4.2	65.7
The middle 60%	5.60	0.32	1.41	7.33	74.3	9.9	69.1
The highest 20%	4.77	0.58	1.92	7.27	64.7	14.9	79.5
13–15 years old							
The lowest 20%	6.36	0.06	1.89	8.31	73.7	1.8	70.5
The middle 60%	6.65	0.37	1.68	8.70	71.3	8.8	64.1
The highest 20%	7.56	0.21	1.92	9.69	79.5	5.1	72.1
16–18 years old							
The lowest 20%	6.13	0.00	1.43	7.56	66.8	0.0	54.2
The middle 60%	7.47	0.15	1.45	9.07	72.7	3.8	48.5
The highest 20%	7.42	0.07	1.75	9.24	69.7	2.1	62.1

For low and middle income families, the increase in public investments can reduce the financial burden on families.[10] For children, this is undoubtedly conducive to reducing the disadvantages in access to education, future employment and socioeconomic inequality that result from lower family income. For parents, increased public investments can free up their time to care for children, giving parents the flexibility to spend their time, extend their labor hours, and increase family income.

Summary

Education equity is an important factor in reducing socioeconomic inequities. This chapter focuses on education equity for children in rural areas and low-income families. This chapter examines the study time of a sample of children aged 3–18 in the 2017 Chinese Time Use Survey data to analyze the current state of educational equity in China. Research found that education equity has been achieved in China's compulsory education, which currently covers the primary and junior high school levels regardless of income levels, mothers' education levels, net enrollment rates of children aged 3–6 in urban and rural households, and time spent in school. Rural families are not guaranteed at the non-compulsory education level, especially the net enrollment and study time of children aged 3–6 from low-income, low-education families. Children's extracurricular tutoring time relies heavily on families' financial investment, and time spent doing homework is associated with parental supervision and tutoring time. Because of the financial commitment and time investment required from families, there is a similar pattern in the amount of time spent on these two out-of-school learning activities for children aged 3–18. Children's out-of-school learning time is generally lower in rural areas, low-income households, and households with low-educated parents than in urban areas, households with high-income levels, and households with well-educated mothers.

In this chapter, we examine educational inequities resulting from differences in children's educational starting points along three dimensions: urban–rural differences, mothers' education levels, and household income. However, there are strong correlations among these three factors: as education increases under the same conditions, one's income also increases; people with high education and high income are relatively concentrated in urban areas because of the difference in production and living conditions between urban and rural areas; the difference in the conditions of education facilities between urban and rural areas leads to inequitable educational outcomes for urban and rural students, widening the income gap and leading to social inequity.

Education investment is a long-term project that consumes a lot of human, financial and material resources. Not only does investment in education increase human capital accumulation, but its externalities also make marginal benefits incremental

[10] C. Gutiérrez, R. Tanaka, "Inequality and Education Decisions in Developing Countries", *Journal of Economic Inequality*, 2009, 7 (1).

and promote the balanced development of the entire regional economy. At present, China's public investment in education and the implementation of various education policies and regulations have effectively reduced the impact of differences in starting points such as urban and rural areas and mothers' education levels and incomes, ensured equality in children's schooling time, and improved educational equity for children in compulsory education. However, extracurricular education for students of non-compulsory education age together with all children still relies heavily on local educational resources and family investments. Therefore, this chapter argues that the country should continue to balance educational development and reduce educational inequities caused by differences in educational starting points. The government should also continue to increase investment in educational infrastructure in rural areas, enhance teacher construction, raise rural teachers' salaries, and provide more educational subsidies to rural, low-education, and low-income families so that children from these families can receive equal education.

Chapter 7
Education Equity in Light of Families' Time Investment in Childcare

As an early investment in human capital, childcare, which includes the care of children's lives, recreation, and education, is critical to promoting children's health, cognitive and non-cognitive development, and thus largely determines the future income and well-being of children.[1] The family production model ultimately combines investment in material and time to maximize family utility.[2] Time investment in childcare impacts early human capital development[3]and is a critical channel leading to the intergenerational transmission of education.[4] Parents' time investment in childcare is positively correlated with parents' education and income levels, and the average participation length of childcare is significantly higher for highly educated and high-income parents than for low-educated and low-income parents, a phenomenon referred to in the literature as the educational gradient and income gradient of childcare time.[5] There are several explanations for this phenomenon in Home Economics, but two of them are generally accepted: one is that childcare is a "luxury" with high-income elasticity, so that as income levels increase, the time devoted to childcare also increases, crowding out time dedicated to other activities (e.g., daily housework and leisure); the other is that childcare, as an investment in human capital, has a higher return on investment for highly educated households than for less educated families, and thus the former are more motivated to invest in childcare than the latter. Whatever the reason, childcare investment is strongly and positively correlated with parents' socioeconomic status, a phenomenon that requires significant attention from policymakers because it can weaken social mobility,

---

[1] Carneiro, Pedro Manuel, and J. J. Heckman, "Human Capital Policy", *Social Science Electronic Publishing*, 2003, 30 (2004).

[2] Becker, Gary S., "A Theory of the Allocation of Time", *Economic Journal*, 1965, 75 (299).

[3] Haveman, Robert and Barbara Wolfe, "The Determinants of Children's Attainments: A Review of Methods and Findings", *Journal of Economic Literature*, 1995, 33 (4).

[4] Datcher-Loury, Linda, "Effects of Mother's Home Time on Children's Schooling", *Review of Economics and Statistics*, 1988, 70 (3).

[5] Guryan, Jonathan, Erik Hust and Melissa Kearney, "Parental Education and Parental Time with Children", *Journal of Economics Perspectives*, 2008, 22 (3).

F. Du et al., *Chinese People's Time Use and Their Quality of Life*,
https://doi.org/10.1007/978-981-99-5526-8_7

challenge notions of social equity based on equal opportunities, and exacerbate socioeconomic inequality.

Adopting data from the 2017 Chinese Time Use Survey, this chapter analyzes the current situation of Chinese families' childcare time investment, and examines whether there is an educational gradient and an income gradient in Chinese families' childcare from the three aspects: urban and rural areas, parents' education level, and family income level. The average participation length and quality of time invested in childcare vary across families, and one of the factors affecting the quality of childcare is the time allocation across different activities. We divide childcare activities into three categories: living care, educational care, and recreational care. Among these, living care includes dressing, feeding, and bathing children. Besides, waiting and transportation activities related to supervising babysitters and picking up and dropping off children are also taken into account. Educational care includes tutoring children with homework and studying and reading with them. Recreational care includes playing and watching TV with children. The higher the percentage of educational care time, the higher the quality of care, given the same total time caring for children. Another factor that affects the quality of care is the role of care providers at different stages of a child's development. Like many countries worldwide, especially developing countries,[6] parents are not the only childcare providers in Chinese families, but grandparents also play an important role. In China, about 32% of children aged 0–3 years are cared for by grandparents[7]; about 58% of grandparents are involved in caring for their grandchildren.[8] During the infant stage, the need for childcare far outweighs the need for educational care, and grandparents may often be more experienced than younger parents. However, by the time children reach the age of receiving formal education, their need for living care decreases and their need for educational care increases. Compared with parents, grandparents are on average less educated, less able to tutor their grandchildren, and may even disagree with their children about their educational philosophy.[9] As parents' education level of preschool-age children in urban China increases, childcare providers gradually shift from grandparent-dominated to parent-dominated.[10] In addition, mothers are responsible for most of the childcare in Chinese families due to the traditional division of labor and gender roles that "men's work centers around outside, while women's

[6] Posadas, Josefina, "Grandparents as Child Care Providers: Factors to Consider When Designing Child Care Policies", *The World Bank Economic Premise*, 2012.

[7] Hangkong Zhang, "The Continuity and Transmutation of Child Care and the Establishment of the 0–3-Year-Old Child Care Service System in China", *Studies in Preschool Education*, 2016 (9).

[8] Fenglian Du, Yingyu Zhang, Xiaoyuan Dong, "The Impact of Child Care Practices on the Labor Force Participation Rate of Women in Urban China", *World Economic Papers*, 2018 (3).

[9] Kun Yue, "Father-Dominated and Grandparent-Supported Parenting Is Conducive to Children's Healthy Growth—Survey on the Status of Grandparent Involvement in Chinese Urban Family Parenting", *Children's Study*, 2018 (1).

[10] Weiwei Li, *Jiefang Daily*, January 7th.

work centers around home". However, fathers' care-giving investment is also essential for developing children's human capital.[11] Studies have shown that as income levels increase, not only does the amount of childcare time mothers spend, but also that of fathers, with parents spending more time caring for children in high-income countries than in low-income countries.[12] This chapter will compare the average participation length of childcare, the composition of care-giving activities, and the identity of caregivers in Chinese families in terms of urban and rural areas, mothers' education level, and per capita household income, respectively.

Who Takes Care of Children?

Based on the United Nations Convention on the Rights of the Child and the reality that children in China largely complete high school education at age 18, we defined children as residents aged 18 and younger. From the data in the 2017 Chinese Time Use Survey, we selected mothers, fathers, grandmothers, and grandfathers living with children aged 0–18 years as our sample. Due to information limitations, we could not distinguish whether they were grandparents or maternal grandparents. Considering that some children also receive care from non-cohabiting grandparents, the data chosen for this chapter underestimate the investment of Chinese grandparents into childcare to some extent.[13] In line with common practice in the childcare literature, information on the main activities performed by the Time Diary fillers on a typical day is used to measure the participation length and rate of the caregivers. It has been noted that childcare can be either a primary or secondary activity, and that much childcare occurs in secondary activities, such as mothers cooking while watching their children or being with their children while engaged in primary activities.[14] The average participation length of childcare as a secondary activity is 1.6 h per day, which is much smaller than that of childcare as a primary activity of 2.59 h per day, so this chapter focuses on the primary activity. The sample analyzed included a total of 4,263 mothers, 4,293 fathers, 2,507 grandmothers, and 2,108 grandfathers.

Table 7.1 reports the urban–rural differences in childcare providers. It can be found that the years of education of urban care providers were significantly higher than those of rural areas. The years of education of urban parents were 2.7–3.0 years higher than those of rural areas, and the years of education of urban grandparents were

[11] Cooksey, Elizabeth and Michelle M. Fondell, "Spending Time with His Kids: Effects of Family Structure on Father's and Children's Lives", *Journal of Marriage and the Family*, 1996, 58 (3).

[12] Guryan, Jonathan, Erik Hust and Melissa Kearney, "Parental Education and Parental Time with Children", *Journal of Economics Perspectives*, 2008, 22 (3).

[13] Du Fenglian et al. estimate that about 14% of children in urban China are cared for by non-cohabiting grandparents. See Fenglian Du, Yingyu Zhang, Xiaoyuan Dong, "The Impact of Child Care Practices on Female Labor Force Participation in Urban China", *World Economic Papers*, 2018 (3).

[14] Folbre, Nancy and Jayoung Yoon, "What is Child Care? Lessons from Time-use Surveys of Major English-speaking Countries", *Review of Economics of the Household*, 2007, 5 (3).

Table 7.1 Personal character of the childcare providers in chinese urban and rural areas

	Age (years old)		Years of education[a] (years)		Employment rate (%)		Paid labor time[b] (hours/day)		Childcare participation rate (%)	
	Rural	Urban	Rural	Urban	Rural	Urban	Rural	Urban	Rural	Urban
Mother	36.1	36.4	7.5	10.5	66.8	69.0	5.07	5.69	36.3	43.3
Father	37.8	38.4	8.4	11.1	87.6	86.0	7.86	8.09	12.1	20.5
Grandmother	60.8	61.5	4.1	6.0	47.0	22.3	2.86	2.06	32.3	38.5
Grandfather	62.2	63.0	6.7	8.3	63.6	40.5	5.40	4.14	15.0	18.3

Note [a] Years of education is converted based on the literacy data, with no school for 0 years, elementary school for 6 years, junior high school for 9 years, high school for 12 years, senior high school/junior college for 12 years, junior college/high vocational school for 15 years, undergraduate for 16 years, master's degree for 19 years, and doctoral degree for 22 years

[b] Paid labor time is the sum of wage labor and family production and operation labor time from the data, the same below

Source 2017 Chinese Time Use Survey and 2017 China Household Finance Survey, the same below

1.6–1.9 years higher than those of rural areas. In both urban and rural areas, fathers and mothers had higher average years of education than grandparents, and men had higher years of education than women. As mentioned earlier, the level of education affects caregivers' parenting philosophy and ability to tutor children in their studies. Also, the labor market participation of care providers affects caregivers' care-giving time. In terms of employment rates, urban mothers were slightly higher than rural mothers, but the employment rates of fathers, grandmothers, and grandfathers were all higher in rural than in urban areas. In terms of paid labor time, urban parents had more paid labor time than rural ones, and rural grandparents had more paid labor time than urban ones. This was because in urban areas, most grandparents withdrew from the labor market when they reached retirement age, and the average paid labor time of grandparents in urban areas decreased; rural pension income was lower, and most rural elderly remained engaged in agricultural production activities after retirement, so the average employment rate and average paid labor time of rural grandparents were higher than those in urban areas. The higher employment rate and paid labor time of rural grandparents may have a negative impact on their time investment in childcare. In terms of care-giving participation rates, urban parents and grandparents had higher participation rates than rural ones. In both urban and rural areas, mothers had much higher childcare participation rates than fathers and grandmothers had much higher childcare participation rates than grandfathers. Childcare participation rates for mothers, fathers, grandmothers, and grandfathers in urban areas were 7.0, 8.4, 6.2, and 3.3% points higher than those in rural areas, respectively. Compared with rural areas, urban parents were somewhat more evenly invested in childcare. Since the education level of urban care providers was generally higher than that of rural families, the difference in childcare participation rates between urban and rural families reflects, to some extent, the educational gradient of care.

Table 7.2 reports the basic profile of childcare providers by mother's education level. Mothers' education level was divided into four categories: elementary school and below, junior high school, senior high school/junior college, and college and above.[15] These four categories of mothers in the sample accounted for 29.8%, 37.6%, 15.7%, and 16.9% of the total sample, respectively. Due to the intergenerational transmission of education, mothers' years of education are positively correlated with the grandparents' years of education. Due to the Forward Matching effect in the marriage market,[16] mothers' years of education are positively correlated with fathers' years of education. Therefore, the years of education of fathers and grandparents are also low in families with low-educated mothers. Both fathers' and grandparents' years of education are relatively high in families with highly educated mothers. The positive correlation between the education level of family caregivers exacerbates the educational gradient in a family's childcare. The employment rates of mothers with college or higher education were significantly higher than those with lower education. Both

[15] There were 707 mothers in the data of this chapter who did not live with the children, at which point we supplemented the mothers' education level with the guardians' education level, using the order of father, grandmother, and grandfather to keep the sample consistent.

[16] Becker G S., *A Theory of Marriage*, 1974.

Table 7.2 Personal character of the childcare providers by mother's education level

	Age (years old)	Years of education[a] (years)	Employment rate (%)	Paid labor time[b] (hours/day)	Childcare participation rate (%)
Elementary school and below (29.8%)					
Mother	38.3	4.5	63.9	5.67	25.1
Father	40.6	7.2	83.5	8.13	9.6
Grandmother	62.7	2.8	36.7	2.77	28.5
Grandfather	64.6	6.0	53.8	4.87	9.4
Junior high school (37.6%)					
Mother	36.0	9.0	67.1	5.35	38.9
Father	37.8	9.5	86.2	7.79	14.3
Grandmother	61.2	5.1	36.5	2.50	34.1
Grandfather	62.1	7.5	54.8	5.10	18.2
High school/junior college (15.7%)					
Mother	34.9	12.0	64.0	4.73	51.3
Father	37.0	11.3	85.8	8.08	71.3
Grandmother	59.7	7.1	33.9	2.04	40.8
Grandfather	61.6	8.6	51.6	4.79	18.5
College and above (16.9%)					
Mother	34.6	15.6	82.3	5.70	55.4
Father	36.1	14.5	93.1	7.74	31.4
Grandmother	59.2	8.2	25.3	2.38	45.5
Grandfather	60.4	9.6	43.2	4.13	22.5

Note The percentage of each degree in the sample is indicated in parentheses after the classification of each degree

mothers' and fathers' childcare participation rates increased with mothers' education levels. Mothers' childcare participation rates increased by 30.3% points and fathers' childcare participation rates increased by 21.8% points for mothers with college education or higher compared to those with primary education or lower. Not only are mother's and father's care participation rates positively correlated with mother's education level, but grandparents in families with mothers with high education also had higher care participation rates than grandparents in families with mothers of low education. For example, grandparents' participation rates were 9.4% and 28.5% for families with elementary school and below, respectively, while they were 22.5% and 45.5% for families with college and above. The childcare participation rate of family members of mothers with low education was much lower than that of family members of mothers with high education, and we see a clear educational gradient in childcare.

Table 7.3 reports basic information on childcare providers by household income level. The sample families were divided into three categories based on quintiles of the distribution of per capita family income across the income distribution in each province: the lowest 20%, the middle 60%, and the highest 20%. It can be found that the level of education of care providers is positively correlated with the level of household income, and the years of education of caregivers in high-income level households are higher than those in low-income households. Also, the employment rates of mothers and fathers in high-income families were higher than those in low-income families. A clear income gradient of care-giving can be seen in childcare participation rates: 34.7%, 16.2%, 28.5%, and 15.8% for mothers, fathers, grandmothers, and grandfathers, respectively, in the lowest 20% of households, and 40.8%, 22.9%, 40.1%, and 17.6%, respectively, in the highest 20% of households.

Tables 7.1, 7.2, and 7.3 show that the participation rates of childcare providers in Chinese families vary considerably between urban and rural families, between families with different levels of maternal education, and between families with different income levels. Were these differences caused by different care needs because of fertility rates, and different numbers of children? To answer this question, Table 7.4 reports the number of children aged 0–18 in different households. The table shows that, relative to urban, high-education and high-income families, rural, low-education and low-income families had more children, while these families had lower care participation rates among care providers. This suggests that the care participation

Table 7.3 Personal character of the childcare providers by household income level

	Age (years old)	Years of education[a] (years)	Employment rate (%)	Paid labor time[b] (hours/day)	Childcare participation rate (%)
The lowest 20%					
Mother	37.1	7.5	63.1	5.26	34.7
Father	39.2	8.2	81.1	7.41	16.2
Grandmother	62.5	3.6	36.5	3.06	28.5
Grandfather	64.7	6.1	50.4	4.48	15.8
The middle 60%					
Mother	36.0	9.1	67.6	5.28	41.5
Father	37.8	9.9	86.8	8.16	15.0
Grandmother	60.6	5.2	35.3	2.35	36.5
Grandfather	61.8	7.6	54.9	5.07	16.6
The highest 20%					
Mother	36.4	12.3	76.9	6.03	40.8
Father	38.4	12.6	92.8	8.13	22.9
Grandmother	61.8	7.2	27.0	2.18	40.1
Grandfather	63.2	9.6	41.9	4.06	17.6

Table 7.4 Average number of children in different families

		Number of children in the family
Urban/rural	Rural	2.03
	Urban	1.58
Mother's education level	Elementary school and below (29.8%)	2.02
	Junior high school (37.6%)	1.81
	High school/junior college (15.7%)	1.59
	College and above (16.9%)	1.35
Per capita household income level	The lowest 20%	2.00
	The middle 60%	1.76
	The highest 20%	1.39

rates and the following analysis of care time somewhat underestimate the educational gradient and income gradient of childcare in Chinese families. This is because with the same total care time, children from families with more children receive less care time on average. Children in rural families and families with low-education, low-income mothers actually receive less care time on average than reported in this chapter.

Inadequate Family Educational Care

This section presents the basic situation of family childcare in China. As shown in Table 7.5, overall, Chinese children aged 0–18 years receive an average of 2.59 h of family care per day, including 1.10 h from mothers, 0.92 h from grandmothers, 0.29 h from fathers, and 0.28 from for grandfathers. Like other countries, women are the primary childcare providers in China, with mothers devoting 3.8 times as much time as fathers and grandmothers devoting 3.3 times as much time as grandfathers. Regarding the type of care, living care, educational care, and recreational care accounted for 71%, 8%, and 21% of total family care time, respectively. Mothers and grandmothers were the main providers of living and recreational care, parents were the main providers of educational care, and grandparents were more likely to substitute for parents in living and recreational care limited by their education level.

In the United States, mothers and fathers spend 2 h and 1 h per day, respectively, on caring for children aged 0–18 years, and educational care accounts for approximately 14% of total care time.[17] The combined care-giving time of Chinese mothers and

[17] Guryan, Jonathan, Erik Hust and Melissa Kearney, "Parental Education and Parental Time with Children", *Journal of Economics Perspectives*, 2008, 22 (3).

Table 7.5 Average participation length of family child care in China. Unit: hours/day

	Living care	Educational care	recreational care	Total care
Mother	0.77	0.12	0.21	1.10
Father	0.17	0.04	0.08	0.29
Grandmother	0.70	0.03	0.19	0.92
Grandfather	0.21	0.01	0.06	0.28
Family total	1.85	0.20	0.54	2.59

grandmothers is similar to that of the mothers from the US, while the combined care-giving time of fathers and grandfathers is only 57% of the care-giving time of the fathers from the US. Mothers from the US spend twice as much time caring as fathers, which is much lower than the care-giving rate of Chinese parents. Total family care-giving time in China is 2.59 h per day, which is lower than the total input of mothers and fathers in US families (3 h), and the proportion of educational care-giving in Chinese families is only about half of the total care-giving time of US families.

The following is a further analysis of the total length of care, the composition of care-giving time, and the roles of caregivers at different stages of a child's development. We divide children's ages into infant and toddler ages of 0–2, preschool ages of 3–6, elementary ages of 7–12, junior high school ages of 13–15, and senior high school ages of 16–18. As children enter different age groups, the family's time commitment to childcare changes accordingly, not only in terms of the division of caregiver labor, but also in the composition of care-giving time. As shown in Table 7.6, the overall average length of family childcare decreased as children grew, with children aged 0–2 years receiving 7.11 h of care per day, compared to only 0.63–0.64 h of family care per day as they entered high school. Mothers were the primary caregivers at all stages of child development, accounting for 35.6–67.2%, while fathers accounted for 9.9–19.7%. Grandparents' contributions were concentrated until children reached secondary school, providing 42–54.5% of care. At the middle and high school levels, the parents' contribution to total family childcare time far exceeded that of the grandparents. It was also found that the amount of time spent in educational care rose and then fell with the age of the child, reaching a peak at 0.27 h per day at the elementary school level.

The Quality of Childcare in Rural Families Is Significantly Lower

This section compares the average length of childcare, the roles of different caregivers, and the composition of care in urban and rural families in China. Childcare in urban and rural families is mainly influenced by three factors: first, public investment and market supply of education in childcare in rural areas still lag behind those in

Table 7.6 Average participation length of childcare and provider contribution by age in Chinese families

Age	Total care time (hours/day)	Educational care (hours/day)	Mother's share (%)	Father's share (%)	Grandparents' share (%)
0–2 years old	7.11	0.13	44.1	10.3	45.6
3–6 years old	3.72	0.16	35.6	9.9	54.5
7–12 years old	1.56	0.27	44.6	13.4	42.0
13–15 years old	0.64	0.19	54.5	19.7	25.8
16–18 years old	0.63	0.10	67.2	15.6	17.2

Note The mother's share is a mother's childcare time percentage of total family care time. Father's share is a father's child care time percentage of total family care time, and grandparent's share is the grandfather's and grandmother's child care time as a percentage of total family care time, the same below

urban areas[18]; second, parents' education and family income levels in rural families are lower than those in urban families, and they need to rely more on society for investment in children's human capital[19]; third, the social atmosphere in rural areas lacks fierce competition and demands for children's academic achievement are as high as that in urban areas.[20]

Figure 7.1 reports the urban–rural differences in childcare providers and care composition. Figure 7.1a shows that in rural areas, total family childcare time averaged 2.73 h per day, with 1.09 h from mothers, 1.12 h from grandmothers, 0.23 h from fathers, and 0.30 h from grandfathers. Compared with rural areas, total family care time was slightly lower in urban areas, averaging 2.48 h per day, with 1.10 h from mothers, 0.34 h from fathers, 0.78 h from grandmothers, and 0.26 h from grandfathers. Comparing urban and rural care providers, it can be seen that urban mothers cared for about the same amount of time as rural mothers, urban fathers cared for more hours than rural fathers, and urban grandparents cared for fewer hours than rural grandparents. Rural mothers spent 4.7 times as much time caring for their fathers, while urban mothers spent 3.2 times as much time caring for their fathers; rural grandparents spent 1.1 times as much time caring for their parents, while urban grandparents spent only 72% of the time caring for their parents.

Figure 7.1b shows that the main component of family childcare is still life care in both rural and urban areas. In particular, rural households spent 0.37 h per day more

[18] Jing Liu, Xiaoyuan Dong, "Maternal Labor Supply, Child Care and Child Health: Evidence from Rural China", *World Economic Papers*, 2011 (4).

[19] Mi'ning Liu, Lutang Li, et al., "Analysis of Child Human Capital Investment Behavior of Rural Families in Western China", *Journal of University of Electronic Science and Technology of China (Social Science Edition)*, 2010 (1).

[20] Tongping Li, "Analysis of Urban–Rural Differences in Family Human Capital Investment", *Society Chinese Journal of Sociology*, 2002 (7).

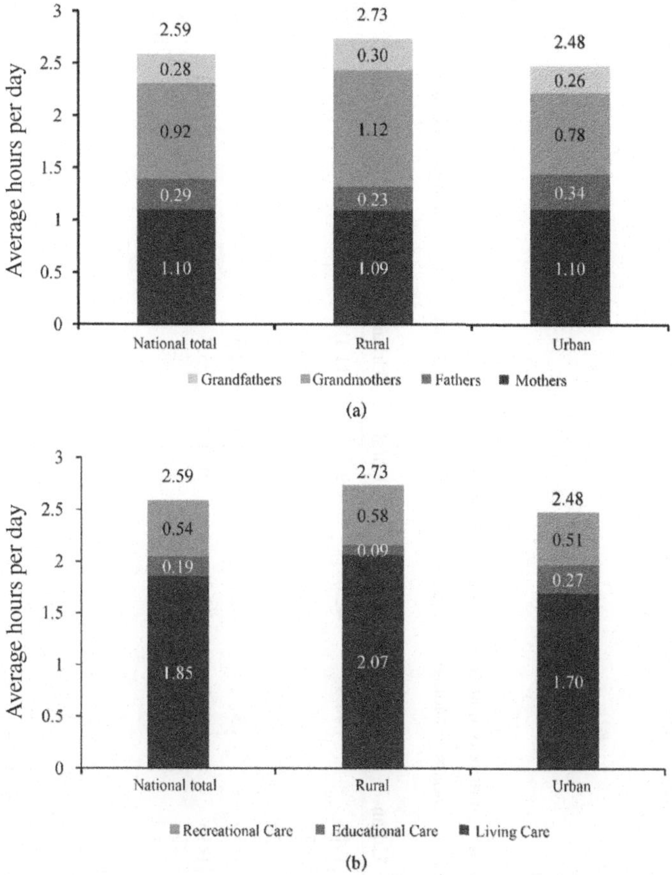

Fig. 7.1 Roles and care composition of childcare providers in urban and rural families in China

on living care than urban households; urban households spent much more time on educational care, about three times more than rural households (0.27 h vs. 0.09 h), and rural households spent slightly more time than urban households on playing with and watching TV (0.58 h vs. 0.51 h).

The difference between urban and rural care providers and educational care time shows that the quality of childcare in rural areas is lower than in towns, which is inseparable from the difference in the education level of urban and rural childcare providers.

Table 7.7 reports the proportion of total care time, educational care time, and parental and grandparental care time to total care time for children of different ages in urban and rural families in China. The table shows that rural families spent significantly more total care time than urban families during the preschool years 0–2 and 3–6, while there was little difference in total care time between the two types of families as they entered the school age. As mentioned earlier, rural families devoted more

Table 7.7 Average participation length of childcare and provider contribution in urban and rural families in China

Age	Total care time (hours/day)		Educational care (hours/day)		Mother's share (%)		Father's share (%)		Grandparents' share (%)	
	Rural	Urban	Rural	Urban	Rural	Urban	Rural	Urban	Rural	Urban
0–2 years old	7.53	6.80	0.07	0.16	46.8	42.0	9.3	11.1	43.9	46.9
3–6 years old	3.37	1.56	0.10	0.22	31.0	39.6	5.7	13.9	63.3	46.5
7–12 years old	1.56	1.57	0.13	0.39	40.7	48.2	9.5	16.3	49.8	35.5
13–15 years old	0.45	0.79	0.06	0.30	37.2	62.2	13.1	22.3	49.7	15.5
16–18 years old	0.67	0.61	0.02	0.16	61.1	72.2	16.4	15.7	22.5	12.1

time to preschool childcare than urban families, in large part because the accessibility of services in rural childcare institutions was significantly lower than in urban areas, and rural families needed to devote more time to caring for infants and preschool-age children. The gap between urban and rural care quality was manifested in three ways: first, as shown in Table 7.7, urban families spent significantly more time on educational care than rural families at all stages of children's development, and the urban–rural gap widened with the growth of children. For age groups of 0–2 years, 3–6 years, 7–12 years, 13–15 years, and 16–18 years, the urban–rural ratio was 2.0, 2.2, 3.0, 5.0, and 8.0, respectively. In terms of family time spent on educational care, rural children were clearly "losing" at the starting line. Second, urban families were more likely to have parents care for their children and less likely to rely on grandparents. Except for the infant and toddler stage of 0–2 years old, when children entered the preschool and primary and secondary education stages of 3–18 years old, urban families had a higher proportion of parents' total family care time than rural families. Especially when children entered the school-age stage, in the elementary school stage of 7–12 years old, the total proportion of rural parents was 50.2%, while that of urban families was 64.5%. In the junior high school stage of 13–15 years old, it was 50.3% in rural areas and 84.5% in urban households; in the senior high school stage of 16–18 years old, it was 77.5% in rural areas and 87.9% in urban areas. Third, the proportion of total family care time spent by urban fathers was by and large significantly higher than that of rural fathers at all ages of children. Up to the middle school level, rural fathers contributed less than 10% and urban fathers contributed more than 10%. In summary, the quality of care received by children in urban areas was higher than that of children in rural areas.

The Educational Gradient of Childcare

This section compares differences in the length and quality of childcare for families with different levels of maternal education. As shown in Fig. 7.2a, overall, the total time spent on childcare increased as the mother's education level increased, e.g., 1.85 h per day for families with mothers with primary education or below, and 3.71 h per day for families with mothers with a college education or above. The number of hours of care-giving in families with high education was almost twice as long as in families with low education. Compared with families in which the mother with an education level of only elementary school or below, families in which the mother's education level was college or higher not only had more total care-giving time, but also had more time invested by each caregiver than the former; the daily care-giving time for mothers, fathers, grandmothers, and grandfathers was 0.69, 0.19, 0.76, and 0.22 h, in the former category respectively, and 1.55, 0.59, 1.16 and 0.41 h in the latter category respectively. As mentioned earlier, the education level of care providers in high-education families, whether parents or grandparents, was higher than that of low-education families, so that childcare provided by high-education families was

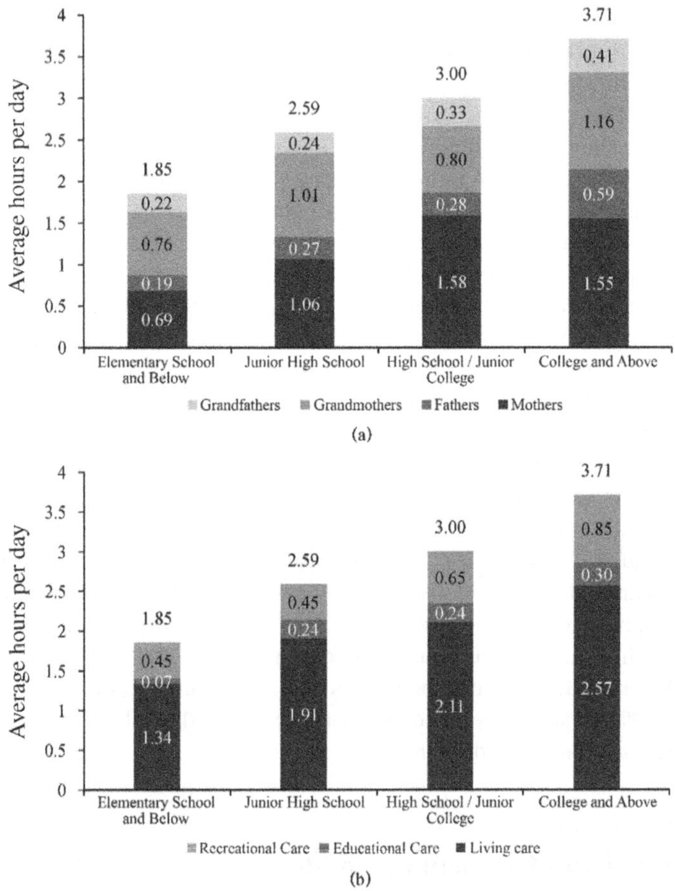

Fig. 7.2 Childcare provider roles and care composition by mother's education level

more than that of low-education families, and possibly higher than that of the latter in quality.

The relative contribution of grandparents and parents also had an impact on the quality of care-giving because the average education level of grandparents was lower than that of parents. Figure 7.2a shows that the proportion of parents in total care-giving time was 48% and 51% in families where mothers had only primary and junior high school education, and 62% and 58% in families where mothers had senior high school/junior college and college and higher education, respectively. The proportion of fathers in childcare was also higher in families with high education than in families with low education. The proportion of fathers' care-giving time was about 10% in families where mothers had only primary and junior high school education and 16% in families where mothers had college and higher education. In terms of parental contribution to childcare alone, the quality of childcare was higher in families with high education than in families with low education.

Figure 7.2b shows that in terms of the composition of care, as the mother's education increased, the amount of time spent in life care increased, but the proportion of the total time spent in family childcare was decreasing. The amount of time spent on educational care was increasing and declined as a proportion of total family childcare time, with the family spending 0.07 h per day on educational care when the mother's education was elementary school and below, and 0.30 h per day when the mother's education is college and above, the latter being 4.3 times more than the former. Families with higher educational attainment devoted significantly less time to the activity of watching TV with their children. For example, the average time spent watching TV with children was 0.11 h for families whose mothers had an elementary school education or below, while it was only 0.04 h for families whose mothers had a college education or more.

Data on household expenditures show that as the mother's education level increased, so did the household's monetary investment in children's education and training. Child education and training expenditures of families with mothers with education levels of elementary school and below, junior high school, senior high school and junior college, and college and above were 5040, 6176, 6094, and 7871 yuan per year, respectively. This indicates that the gap in childcare and education investment among families with mothers of different education levels was not only in terms of time investment but also in terms of education expenditure. Compared to families with low-educated mothers, children in families with high education had more opportunities to attend tutoring classes and tutors. Low-educated mothers not only had limited ability to tutor their children themselves, but also could not afford to compensate for their own shortcomings by purchasing specialized services.

Table 7.8 reports the differences in total childcare hours, educational care hours, and parental and grandparental care hours as a proportion of total family care hours for families with different mothers' education levels for each age group of children. Because of the further decomposition of the five child age groups into four educational categories, some of which had fewer observations. There were some child age groups in which mothers' education level and care-giving time did not consistently show a positive association. As mothers' education level increased during the 3–15 years' stage, the family's total care time and time spent on educational care would also increase. In addition, the proportion of total family care time spent by both mothers and fathers increased with maternal education at almost all ages of children; fathers in families with mothers with college or higher education contributed more to childcare than other types of families (except at the 13–15 years' stage). The positive correlation between mothers' education and fathers' contribution to childcare may be due to two reasons. First, because of the Forward Matching effect of marriage, and fathers with higher education are more likely to spend more time on childcare because they understand the importance of fathers' involvement in childcare. Second, mothers with higher education had higher incomes and therefore had more bargaining power in the division of labor within the household. The childcare "deficit" was most severe for mothers with only elementary school education or below, except for the

Table 7.8 Average participation length of childcare and provider contribution by mother's education level

	Total care time (hours/day)	Educational care (hours/day)	Mother's share (%)	Father's share (%)	Grandparents' share (%)
0–2 years old					
Elementary school and below	5.97	0.12	41.1	8.0	50.9
Junior high school	7.98	0.12	41.5	9.0	49.5
High school/junior college	6.86	0.18	56.2	7.8	36.0
College and above	7.18	0.11	40.1	12.9	45.0
3–6 years old					
Elementary school and below	3.27	0.05	28.5	9.4	62.1
Junior high school	3.65	0.19	33.3	8.3	58.4
High school/junior college	4.10	0.25	43.7	7.3	49.0
College and above	4.20	0.21	39.3	15.9	44.8
7–12 year old					
Elementary school and below	1.48	0.11	34.8	13.6	48.6
Junior high school	1.65	0.30	45.1	10.8	44.1
High school/junior college	1.50	0.35	56.2	15.1	28.7
College and above	1.64	0.63	51.8	18.9	29.3
13–15 years old					
Elementary school and below	0.42	0.04	43.8	11.5	44.7
Junior high school	0.78	0.29	52.4	25.4	22.2
High school/junior college	0.69	0.15	64.3	18.7	17.0
College and above	0.93	0.47	73.8	14.4	11.8

(continued)

Table 7.8 (continued)

	Total care time (hours/day)	Educational care (hours/day)	Mother's share (%)	Father's share (%)	Grandparents' share (%)
16–18 years old					
Elementary school and below	0.41	0.01	70.6	0.5	28.9
Junior high school	0.86	0.20	65.9	19.6	14.5
High school/junior college	0.75	0.13	85.3	14.6	0.1
College and above	0.48	0.08	31.9	48.1	20.0

0–2-year age group. These families had the lowest total care time and educational care time compared to families with other levels of education at all child ages, and grandparents had the highest proportion of total care time.

The Income Gradient of Childcare

Figure 7.3 demonstrates the differences in the amount of time spent on childcare per day by families at different income levels. As shown in Fig. 7.3a, total childcare time was 2.48 h per day for low-income families, 2.67 h per day for middle-income families, and 2.38 h per day for high-income families, with high-income families spending the least amount of time on childcare, probably because this group of families had a greater ability to pay for childcare from the market, replacing the intra-household provision of childcare. Nonetheless, parental care time was higher in high-income households than in middle- and low-income households, and, like high-education households, high-income households preferred parents to care for their own children rather than rely on grandparents, while high-income fathers contributed more to childcare than middle- and low-income households. The percentage of total family care time spent by parents was 66% in high-income families, 52% in middle-income families, and 53% in low-income families; the percentage of total family care time spent by fathers was 18%, 9%, and 15%, respectively. Fathers' care-giving hours and contributions were the lowest in middle-income families among the three income levels.

Figure 7.3b shows the composition of time spent on care-giving for families at different income levels. It can be seen that the amount of time spent on educational care increased with family income, with high-income families spending 1.5 times more total time on educational care than middle-income families and 1.8 times more than low-income families. The data also show that high- and middle-income families

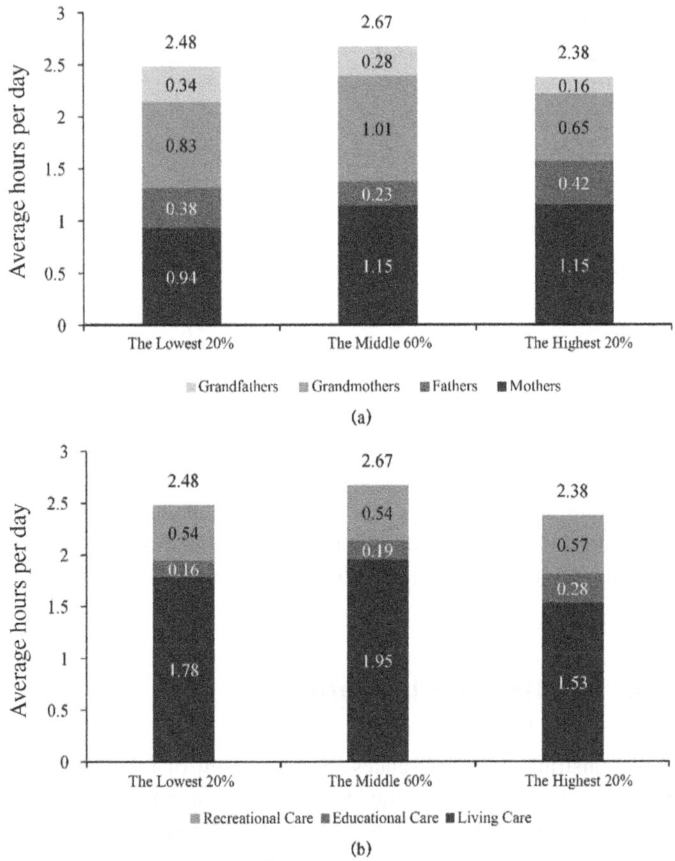

Fig. 7.3 Childcare provider roles and care composition by family income level

spent less time watching TV with their children than low-income families, with 0.04, 0.06, and 0.10 h per day for the three types of families, respectively.

The data on household expenditures show that families with high-income levels also spent more money on education and training. High-income households spent an average of 8,825 yuan per year on their children's education and training, compared to 5,913 yuan for middle-income households and 4,738 yuan for low-income households, with high-income households spending 1.5 times more than middle-income households and 1.9 times more than low-income households. Chinese families' spending on their children's education also reflects the income gradient phenomenon.

Table 7.9 reports differences in total childcare hours, educational care hours, and parental and grandparental care hours as a proportion of total family care hours for families at different income levels for each age group of children. Similar to the effect of the mother's education, the five age groups are further decomposed into three income categories, some of which had fewer observations, so that family income level

Table 7.9 Average participation length of childcare and provider contribution by family income level

Household income level	Total care time (hours/day)	Educational care (hours/day)	Mother's share (%)	Father's share (%)	Grandparents' share (%)
0–2 years old					
The lowest 20%	7.72	0.07	42.8	12.7	44.5
The middle 60%	7.16	0.14	44.2	8.3	47.5
The highest 20%	6.26	0.12	45.1	15.9	39.0
3–6 years old					
The lowest 20%	3.80	0.16	30.8	11.8	57.4
The middle 60%	3.80	0.15	34.9	8.7	56.4
The highest 20%	3.27	0.27	49.5	14.5	36.0
7–12 year old					
The lowest 20%	1.51	0.19	35.3	21.9	42.8
The middle 60%	1.58	0.28	46.9	8.7	44.4
The highest 20%	1.59	0.43	45.6	43.7	10.7
13–15 years old					
The lowest 20%	0.62	0.21	52.1	21.4	26.5
The middle 60%	0.67	0.14	58.9	12.7	28.4
The highest 20%	0.65	0.40	45.6	43.7	10.7
16–18 years old					
The lowest 20%	0.79	0.14	54.0	25.3	20.7
The middle 60%	0.61	0.12	74.9	9.2	15.9
The highest 20%	0.47	0.04	60.7	30.2	9.1

and care-giving time did not consistently show a positive correlation at the individual child's age. However, at the preschool, elementary, and junior high school ages of 3–15, educational care-giving time was significantly higher for high-income families than for low-income families. At the 0–13 years' stage, the proportion of mother's care time was higher in high-income families than in middle- and low-income families, and at the 13–18 years' stage, the proportion of father's care time was higher in high-income families than in middle- and low-income families. Notably, fathers in middle-income families had the shortest care-giving time and the lowest relative contribution, which was present at all ages of the child's life. The fact that fathers in middle-income households spent less time caring than low-income households might be due to the fact that middle-income households had a stronger desire to improve the economic status of their families and, therefore, fathers devoted more time to paid work, crowding out time for childcare. The share of grandparental care in total care was lower in high-income families than in middle- and low-income families at all ages of children, and high-income families were less dependent on grandparental care.

Summary

This chapter analyzes the differences in childcare time investment among Chinese families in terms of urban and rural areas, mothers' education level, and family income level. By comparing the differences in total family childcare time, educational care time, and the contributions of different care providers, we examine whether there is an educational gradient and an income gradient in family childcare in China.

For children aged 0–18 years overall, childcare in Chinese families is provided primarily by mothers and grandmothers, who contribute 42% and 36% of total family care time, respectively. Compared to US mothers and fathers, Chinese mothers and fathers spend less time caring for children, only 55% and 29% of the former, respectively; the gap between Chinese parents' childcare inputs is even greater, with Chinese mothers spending 3.8 times more time caring for children than fathers[21] and US mothers spending 2.0 times more time caring for children than fathers.

From the perspective of childcare providers, urban parents and grandparents have longer years of education than rural parents. Rural mothers have lower employment rates than urban mothers. Both fathers and grandparents have higher employment rates in rural than in urban areas, and urban family members have higher participation rates in childcare than rural families.

From an urban–rural perspective, for children aged 0–18 as a whole, the total care time of rural families is slightly higher than that of urban families, and urban families have an advantage over rural families in terms of the quality of care investment. This

[21] According to the China Family Development Report 2015, China shows a smaller family size and diverse family types, with fathers playing a more limited role and role in the care and education of children.

is evident in three ways. First, urban families spend more time on educational care than rural families at all stages of children's development, and the gap between the two increases with the age of children. In general, urban families spend three times more time on child education and care than rural families. Second, urban families rely less on grandparental care than rural families, except for the 0–2-year-old infant and toddler stage. Third, urban fathers devoted more time to care-giving than rural fathers, 1.5 times more than the latter. Urban fathers contribute more to childcare than rural fathers, except at the 16–18-year-old stage. Since the education level of childcare providers in urban households is higher than that in rural households, the urban–rural difference in childcare quality reflects to some extent the phenomenon of the educational gradient.

In terms of the mother's education level, as the mother's education level increases, parental childcare time increases, grandparental childcare time decreases, and families spend more time on child education care. At the same time, the amount of money families spend on education and training for their children also increases. Families with mothers with an education of elementary school or below have the largest childcare deficit, spending less time on total care and less time on educational care, and relying the most on grandparents for care. These families not only have limited ability to tutor their children, but also cannot afford to purchase professional services to compensate for this deficit.

In terms of family income level, although the total care time of high-income families is lower than that of low- and middle-income families, high-income families invest the most time in educational care, spend the most on education and training, spend the most time on father care, and rely the least on grandparent care. Fathers in middle-income level families spend the least time in childcare compared to low-income and high-income families, at only 55% of the amount spent in high-income families.

In summary, the education gradient and income gradient of childcare time in Chinese families are obvious, and there is an apparent "care deficit" in rural families, low-education and low-income families. The "care deficit" is evident in rural families, low-education and low-income families. Because of the law of increasing returns on human capital investment, gaps in early childhood development, if not intervened in a timely manner, will continue to widen with age and family investment, depriving children from lower socioeconomic families of equal opportunities to compete in the labor market. The education gradient and income gradient in childcare need to be of great concern to policymakers. For some rural families, low-education and low-income families, governments at all levels should take effective interventions to increase the supply of public education, so that parents who are unable to tutor their children can compensate for their lack of capacity through preschools, schools and social services. The National Development Plan for Children in Poor Areas from 2014 to 2020 proposes to adhere to the basic policy of early childhood development intervention. The China Child Development Report 2017: Anti-Poverty and Early Childhood Development incorporates early childhood development into the national anti-poverty strategy and proposes the establishment of an early childhood development system in poor areas with full intervention and comprehensive protection.

These initiatives can help close the "care deficit" of families in poor areas and break the intergenerational transmission of poverty. If proven effective, these interventions should be extended to non-poor, low-education and low-income families to achieve social equity in education on a larger scale.

Improving the quality of family childcare investment also need to encourage Chinese fathers to become more involved in childcare[22] and to share childcare responsibilities with mothers. Grandparents play an important role in childcare for rural families, low-education and low-income families, and their education level is generally lower than that of the child's parents; they can be trained in childcare to understand contemporary educational concepts better, recognize the importance of educational care, and acquire new parenting techniques.[23]

---

[22] Studies have found that fathers play an important role in children's character building, intellectual development and self-discipline.

[23] In recent years, some well-known educational institutions in Guangzhou and Shanghai have launched "parenting classes" in which 80% of the students are not parents, but grandparents, who learn new parenting knowledge and early childhood development concepts to relieve the pressure of living in urban dual-income families. The project is jointly promoted by the National Health and Family Planning Commission and the Rural Education Action Program (REAP, a joint project of the Institute of Experimental Economics in Education of Shaanxi Normal University, the Agricultural Policy Research Center of the Chinese Academy of Sciences, and Stanford University). The early infant and toddler development project, called Parenting the Future, conducts experiment in early infant and toddler development interventions in rural areas. The project aims to raise awareness among rural parents about proper parenting by training former grassroots family planning cadres to become "parenting teachers" to provide counseling to guardians of infants and toddlers aged 0–3 in rural families.

Chapter 8
Are Children Sleep-Deprived?

Sufficient sleep positively impacts the healthy development of children and adolescents physically and mentally. In contrast, lack of sleep can lead to low energy, poor abstract thinking and memory, emotional disturbance, drug abuse and even impairment of growth and development.[1] In addition, sleep duration is associated with smoking, alcohol consumption, drug abuse, and injuries among children and adolescents.[2] Sleep deprivation also increases the risk of obesity, diabetes, cardiovascular diseases, infectious diseases, etc.[3] Therefore, the adequacy of sleep among children and adolescents is of crucial importance for their healthy growth, and further answers the sufficiency of sleep among children and adolescents in China based on the results of nationally representative basic data analysis, which support the development of health education and intervention measures related to children and adolescents.

Based on this, this chapter analyzes the sleep status of Chinese children and adolescents using data from the 2017 Chinese Time Use Survey, focusing on answering the following questions: do Chinese children and adolescents get enough sleep? What structural characteristics do sleep-deprived children and adolescents have? What factors influence children's and adolescents' sleep?

Focusing on the above questions, firstly, this chapter reports the basic situation of sleep among children and adolescents in China; secondly, it makes international and cross-period comparisons of sleep among children and adolescents; thirdly, it analyzes factors that may affect sleep among children and adolescents; and finally, summarizes the full text.

---

[1] Azadbakht L., Kelishadi R., Khodarahmi M., "The Association of Sleep Duration and Cardio Metabolic Risk Factors in A National Sample of Children and Adolescents: The CASPIAN III Study", *Nutrition*, 2013, 29 (9).

[2] Adolescent Sleep Working Group, Committee on Adolescents, Council on School Health, "School Start Times for Adolescents", *Am Academy Pediatrics*, 2014, 134 (3).

[3] Keyes K. M., Maslowsky J., Hamilton A, "The Great Sleep Recession: Changes in Sleep Duration Among US Adolescents", *Pediatrics*, 2015, 135 (3).

F. Du et al., *Chinese People's Time Use and Their Quality of Life*,
https://doi.org/10.1007/978-981-99-5526-8_8

Basic Information on Children and Adolescents' Sleep

In the 2017 Chinese Time Use Survey, a total of 3,149 samples of children and adolescent students were obtained (see Table 8.1 for details), including 1,706 children aged 6–11 years, accounting for 54.2%; 791 adolescents aged 12–14 years, accounting for 25.1%; 652 adolescents aged 15–17 years, accounting for 20.7%. In the total sample, there were 1,672 boys (53.1%) and 1,477 girls (46.9%).

According to the *Health Requirements of Daily Learning Time for Secondary and Elementary School Students* issued by the National Health and Family Planning Commission on May 1st, 2013, primary school students should not sleep less than 10 h per day, middle school students should not sleep less than 9 h per day, and high school students should not sleep less than 8 h per day. Taking this as a reference, the data analysis on the sleep status of children and adolescents in the 2017 Chinese Time Use Survey shows (see Table 8.2) that if naps and night sleep were combined, the average daily sleep duration of Chinese children aged 6–11 was above 10 h, and adolescents aged 12–17 slept more than 9 h per day. In all age groups, the sleep duration was higher than the recommended standard by the National Health and Family Planning Commission.

Judging from the sleep deprivation rate of the sample, even including nap time, the problem of sleep deprivation among children and adolescents was still considerable, with 31.0, 22.2, and 20.2% for students aged 6–11, 12–14, and 15–17 years old, respectively. As age increased, the rate of sleep deprivation reporting decreased (see Table 8.3).

Referring to international statistical standards, the sleep duration of children and adolescents is limited to nighttime sleep only. In this regard, the sleep deprivation rate of this group climbed rapidly (see Table 8.4). The average daily nighttime sleep duration of children aged 6–11 in China was below 10 h, which was lower than the recommended standard of the National Health and Family Planning Commission. The problem of sleep deprivation among children was evident in urban and rural areas, which needed urgent attention. The daily nighttime sleep duration of adolescents aged 12–14 was around 9 h, and the average sleep duration of adolescents in urban areas was lower than the recommended standard of the National Health and Family

Table 8.1 Sample distribution of children and adolescents in the 2017 Chinese Time Use Survey Unit: person

Sample	Urban		Rural		Total
	Boys	Girls	Boys	Girls	
6–11 years old	528	500	369	309	1706
12–14 years old	261	203	172	155	791
15–17 years old	224	207	118	103	652
Total	1013	910	659	567	3149

Source The 2017 Chinese Time Use Survey, the same below

Table 8.2 Sleep duration statistics of in-school students in China (including naps) Unit: hours/day

People		National total	Urban	Rural
All sample	Total	10.14	10.11	10.17
	Boys	10.09	10.07	10.11
	Girls	10.20	10.17	10.23
6–11 years old	Total	10.67	10.81	10.51
	Boys	10.66	10.77	10.53
	Girls	10.69	10.86	10.48
12–14 years old	Total	9.85	9.76	9.98
	Boys	9.81	9.71	9.94
	Girls	9.89	9.80	10.04
15–17 years old	Total	9.25	9.09	9.50
	Boys	9.15	9.05	9.30
	Girls	9.38	9.15	9.78

Table 8.3 Sleep deprivation rate (including naps) among children and adolescents aged 6–17 years in China in 2017 unit: %

Gender and age		National total	Urban	Rural
Gender	Male	26.1	24.9	27.8
	Female	26.6	26.9	26.2
Age	6–11	31.0	27.2	35.7
	12–14	22.2	24.5	18.8
	15–17	20.2	24.3	13.9

Planning Commission. The nighttime sleep duration of adolescents aged 15–17 was more than 8 h per day.

Judging from the sleep deprivation rate of the sample (see Table 8.5), if the nap was not included, the sleep deprivation rate of children and adolescents aged 6–17 was as high as about 50%. Moreover, the sleep deprivation rate of children and adolescents decreased as age increased. The sleep deprivation rates were 54.7, 43.7, and 41.7% for students aged 6–11, 12–14, and 15–17, respectively.[4]

[4] The newly released *China Compulsory Education Quality Monitoring Report* shows that 30.7% of fourth graders slept 10 h or more, or 69.3% of sleep deprivation; 16.6% of eighth graders slept 9 h or more, or 83.4% of sleep deprivation. The results differed because of the sample selected and the survey method.

Table 8.4 Sleep duration statistics of in-school students in China (excluding naps) Unit: hours/day

People		National total	Urban	Rural
All sample	Total	9.24	9.21	9.29
	Boys	9.21	9.15	9.28
	Girls	9.28	9.27	9.30
6–11 years old	Total	9.79	9.86	9.70
	Boys	9.79	9.81	9.76
	Girls	9.79	9.91	9.63
12–14 years old	Total	9.00	8.92	9.12
	Boys	8.98	8.94	9.03
	Girls	9.03	8.89	9.24
15–17 years old	Total	8.29	8.21	8.41
	Boys	8.19	8.07	8.36
	Girls	8.41	8.41	8.49

Table 8.5 Sleep deprivation rate among children and adolescents aged 6–17 years in China in 2017 (excluding naps) Unit: %

Gender and age		National total	Urban	Rural
Gender	Male	48.3	48.4	48.2
	Female	49.9	49.0	51.1
Age	6–11	54.7	52.0	58.0
	12–14	43.7	45.4	41.4
	15–17	41.7	45.3	36.1

International Comparison of Sleep in Children and Adolescents

Sleep deprivation among children and adolescents has become a widespread and international health problem. The National Sleep Foundation of the U.S. has given sleep duration recommendations for different age groups based on expert research results, precisely 9–11 h of sleep per day for children aged 6–13 years old and 8–10 h of sleep per day for adolescents aged 14–17.[5] Table 8.6 compares and analyzes the average sleep duration of children and adolescents aged 4–16 years in China and the U.S. in Table 8.6, the average sleep duration of Chinese school-age children is lower than that of American children at all stages without counting naps, which indicates that the sleep situation of Chinese children is not optimistic.

[5] Knutson K. L., Lauderadale D. S., "Sleep Duration and Overweight in Adolescents: Self-reported Sleep Hours Versus Time Diaries", *Pediatrics*, 2017, 119 (5).

Table 8.6 Comparison of sleep duration of children and adolescents aged 4–16 years between China and the United States Unit: hours/day

	4 years old	6 years old	8 years old	10 years old	12 years old	14 years old	16 years old
China	9.93	9.90	9.68	9.58	9.45	8.77	8.52
The US	10.92	10.39	10.36	9.82	9.58	9.22	9.04

Studies show that children aged 12–14 years in the UK sleep 9.5 h per day and adolescents aged 15–17 years sleep 9.08 h per day.[6] In Australia, children aged 12–14 all sleep more than 9 h per day, and children aged 15–17 all sleep more than 8 h per day.[7] In Canada, adolescents aged 6–17 slept 9.64 h per day.[8] In Italy, children aged 7–10 years sleep 9.50 h per day and those aged 10–14 sleep 9.00 h per day.[9] In India, children aged 10–15 years sleep 9.09 h per day.[10] The average daily sleep duration for children and adolescents aged 6–17 in China is 9.24 h, which is lower than the sleep duration of children in the corresponding age group in the United States and the United Kingdom.[11]

Cross-Period Comparison of Sleep of Children and Adolescents

To further elucidate the changes in the sleep of Chinese children and adolescents over time, the author conducted a cross-period comparison of sleep duration in 2012 and 2017, to observe whether the sleep duration of Chinese children and adolescents has improved in the longitudinal dimension. The sleep data in 2012 were obtained from the monitoring data of Chinese residents' nutrition and health status conducted by Song Chao et al. from 2010 to 2012. The data were collected using multistage stratified cluster random sampling proportional to the population. In the first stage, a total of 150 counties were selected as monitoring sites from four types of areas; in the

[6] Short S., "Adolescents' Health and Well-being in the United Kingdom", *Loisir et Société/Society and Leisure*, 2005, 28 (2).

[7] Olds T., Mather C., Blunden S., "Normative Data on the Sleep Habits of Australian Children and Adolescents", *Sleep*, 2010, 33 (10).

[8] Carson V., Tremblay M. S., Chaput J. P., "Associations between Sleep Duration, Sedentary Time, Physical Activity, and Health Indicators among Canadian Children and Youth Using Compositional Analyses", *Apply Physiology Nutria Metab*, 2016, 41 (6).

[9] Brambilla P., Giussani M., Pasinato A., "Sleep Habits and Pattern in 1–14 Years Old Children and Relationship with Video Devices Use and Evening and Night Activities", *Italy Journal of Pediatric*, 2017, 43.

[10] Bapat R., Van Geel M., Vedder P., "Socio-economic Status, Time Spending, and Sleep Duration in Indian Children and Adolescents", *Journal of Child Family Study*, 2017, 26 (1).

[11] To increase comparability, the sleep duration of Chinese children and adolescents here does not include naptime.

Table 8.7 Daily sleep duration for children and adolescents aged 6–17 years in China in 2012 and 2017 Unit: hours/day

Gender and age		2012			2017			Change		
		National total	Urban	Rural	National total	Urban	Rural	National total	Urban	Rural
Gender	Male	8.47	7.44	8.49	10.09	10.07	10.11	+1.62	+1.63	+1.62
	Female	8.44	7.41	8.46	10.2	10.17	10.23	+1.76	+1.76	+1.77
Age	6–11	8.95	7.99	8.92	10.67	10.81	10.51	+1.72	+1.82	+1.59
	12–14	8.35	8.26	8.43	9.85	9.76	9.98	+1.50	+1.50	+1.55
	15–17	7.73	7.63	7.82	9.25	9.09	9.50	+1.52	+1.46	+1.68

Note The *Change* was calculated by minus the 2012 data from the 2017 data, the same below

second stage, 6 villages were chosen equally spaced using a method proportional to the population; in the third stage, 75 households were randomly selected in each of the selected villages. The health data of children and adolescents aged 6–17 years were collected through questionnaires. 38,744 children and adolescents aged 6–17 years in China were surveyed, of which 19,631 (50.67%) were male and 19,113 (49.33%) were female. There were 19,471 urban students, accounting for 50.26%, and 19,273 rural students, accounting for 49.74%.[12] To increase comparability, referring to the 2012 definition, we defined sleep duration as the sum of sleep time in the afternoon and at night, excluding napping and rest between classes or activities. Sleep deprivation was defined as less than 10 h of sleep per day for elementary school students, less than 9 h for junior high school students, and less than 8 h for senior high school students.

The statistical results show that, overall, there was a significant improvement in sleep among Chinese children and adolescents in 2017 compared with 2012, and this improvement is reflected in: first, a substantial increase in the average duration of sleep; and second, a significant decrease in the rate of sleep deprivation.

A Comparison of Sleep Duration Across Time

In 2012, the average daily sleep duration of children and adolescents aged 6–17 years in China was 8.45 h, with 8.95 h for 6–11 years, 8.35 h for 12–14 years, and 7.73 h for 15–17 years. It can be seen that as the age group grows, the sleep duration is on a decreasing trend. By 2017, the average sleep duration of children and adolescents aged 6–17 years in China reached 10.14 h, with an increase of more than one hour in all age groups compared to 2012 (see Table 8.7).

[12] Chao Song, Weiyan Gong, Caitui Ding, Yan Zhang, Fan Yuan, Ailing Liu, "Sleep Status of Children and Adolescents Aged 6–17 Years in China from 2010–2012", *Chinese Journal of School Health*, 2017 (9).

Table 8.8 Sleep deprivation rates among children and adolescents aged 6–17 years in China in 2012 and 2017 Unit: %

Gender and Age		2012			2017			Change		
		National Total	Urban	Rural	National Total	Urban	Rural	National Total	Urban	Rural
Gender	Male	69.7	71.9	69.3	26.1	24.9	27.8	−43.6	−47.0	−41.5
	Female	69.8	72.2	69.6	26.6	26.9	26.2	−43.2	−45.3	−43.4
Age	6–11	74.0	79.6	73.8	31.0	27.2	35.7	−43.0	−52.4	−38.1
	12–14	71.2	71.1	68.3	22.2	24.5	18.8	−49.0	−46.6	−49.5
	15–17	61.7	60.5	63.5	20.2	24.3	13.9	−41.5	−36.2	−49.6

Comparison of Sleep Deprivation Rates Across Time

Table 8.8 reports the sleep deprivation rates of children and adolescents aged 6–17 years in China in 2012 and 2017. In 2012, the average daily sleep deprivation rate of children and adolescents aged 6–17 years in China was 69.8%, slightly lower in rural areas than in urban areas, and basically the same for boys and girls (69.7, 69.8%). Children aged 6–11 years had the highest sleep deprivation rate, and the rate of sleep deprivation tended to decrease as age increased. Compared with the situation in 2012, the sleep deprivation rate of Chinese children and adolescents decreased by more than 40% points on average in 2017, indicating that sleep deprivation among Chinese children and adolescents has improved significantly.

Compared with 2012, the sleep situation of children and adolescents in 2017 was significantly better. So, what are the reasons behind this result? It is generally believed that children's sleep duration is influenced by various factors, such as time use, especially moderate-to-intense exercise, sedentary time, and video time, in addition to the external environment.[13] However, none of these reasons may be sufficient to reveal the dramatic change in sleep duration compared to 2012, because it is difficult to see a dramatic change in the time use of children and adolescents in a short period of time without a large-scale intervention by external forces.

The author speculates that the most likely reason is the promotion of national policies to reduce the burden, especially after the introduction of the *National Medium- and Long-term Education Reform and Development Plan (2010–2020)*, the central and local governments have introduced various initiatives to reduce the burden of children and adolescents, mainly including: promulgating policies to reduce the burden of schoolwork, postponing the morning school hours, changing school evaluation indicators. These measures have had a positive effect on improving the sleep of children and adolescents.[14]

[13] Chaput J. P., Dutil C., "Lack of Sleep as a Contributor to Obesity in Adolescents: Impacts on Eating and Activity Behaviors", *International Journal of Behavior Nutrition Physics Act*, 2016, 13 (1).

[14] Wenhe Li, "Research on the Classwork Burden of Primary School Students in Shanghai", Shanghai Normal University, 2017; Huimin Hu, Yuxin Yin, "The Journey and Reflections on

However, it should be noted that despite this, the sleep deprivation rate is still considerable, reaching 31.0 and 22.2% for children aged 6–11 and 12–14, respectively, and about 20% for children aged 15–17. Based on this result, the problem of sleep deprivation among Chinese children and adolescents still needs to be taken seriously.

Analysis of Factors Influencing Sleep of Children and Adolescents

Structural Characteristics of the Sleep-Deprived

The following part analyzes which groups are in a sleep-deprived state, or what characteristics of sleep-deprived children and adolescents have, a question that can be addressed to narrow the targeting of policy interventions and improve their targeting and effectiveness.

Tables 8.9 and 8.10 report the proportion of sleep-deprived children and adolescents with different grades. The school performance here was self-rated by parents or students and was divided into three categories: good, upper middle and moderate and below. As can be seen from the statistics in the tables, the differences in sleep deprivation rates among the three stages of the sample are very pronounced when naptime is included. For children aged 6–11 years, samples with upper middle and lower grades in urban areas were more likely to be sleep deprived than those with good grades; similarly, in rural areas, samples with middle and lower grades were more likely to be sleep deprived. For children and adolescents aged 12–14 years, the overall sleep deprivation rate decreased from the 6–11-year-old sample, but was still substantial. For the 15–17-year-old sample, the rate of sleep deprivation was higher for high-achieving students in urban areas than for other students, while the opposite was true in rural areas, possibly due to the greater academic pressure on high school seniors.

If excluding nap time, the statistics in Table 8.10 show that urban boys and rural children aged 6–11 years were more likely to be sleep deprived the worse their grades were, and there was no significant difference in sleep deprivation rates among urban girls with different grades. Among adolescents aged 12–14, boys with moderate grades and below were most likely to be sleep deprived, and urban and rural girls with upper middle grades were most likely to be sleep deprived. Urban adolescents aged 15–17 with good grades had the highest rate of sleep deprivation and it decreased with declining grades.

This finding raises the possibility that, from a child-adolescent developmental perspective, poor academic performance, long homework time and sleep deprivation

Reducing the Classwork Burden of Primary and Secondary Schools in China", *Global Education*, 2015, (44).

Table 8.9 Percentage of sleep deprivation (including naps) among adolescents of children with different grades Unit: %

People		Sleep deprivation proportion			
		Urban		Rural	
Age	Grades	Boys	Girls	Boys	Girls
6–11 years old	Good	23.8	24.3	25.8	26.0
	Upper middle	31.3	25.6	32.3	36.1
	Moderate and below	29.9	27.1	39.9	45.3
12–14 years old	Good	10.6	32.1	16.0	6.4
	Upper middle	17.8	25.2	7.6	27.0
	Moderate and below	17.9	42.3	25.1	18.9
15–17 years old	Good	41.3	39.2	2.5	6.0
	Upper middle	34.4	20.7	20.2	7.3
	Moderate and below	15.1	17.1	18.9	9.8

Table 8.10 Prevalence of sleep deprivation among adolescents with different grades (excluding naps) Unit: %

People		Sleep deprivation proportion			
		Urban		Rural	
Age	Grades	Boys	Girls	Boys	Girls
6–11 years old	Good	43.5	51.6	51.9	58.0
	Upper middle	52.9	50.4	56.0	60.9
	Moderate and below	58.9	51.3	56.9	63.6
12–14 years old	Good	32.7	46.6	39.7	33.3
	Upper middle	32.7	58.3	23.7	45.3
	Moderate and below	47.1	48.6	47.3	43.9
15–17 years old	Good	67.6	54.6	47.5	38.1
	Upper middle	46.6	49.0	52.8	25.5
	Moderate and below	41.9	35.7	29.0	36.1

may form a vicious cycle: poor academic performance requires intensive study and more homework, which in turn leads to insufficient sleep duration, and sleep deprivation leads to low energy, reduced abstract thinking and memory in children, thus affecting academic performance. This determination will be further tested in the next section.

Factors Influencing Sleep Deprivation

Data from the 2017 Chinese Time Use Survey show that the most important factor affecting children and adolescents' sleep is the time spent doing homework. Too much time spent doing homework is currently the most important cause of sleep deprivation among Chinese children and adolescents. We provide a specific analysis below. Tables 8.11 and 8.12 report the main bedtime activities of children and adolescents. The statistical results show that, regardless of whether naps are included or not, by comparing the bedtime activities of the two groups of sleep-sufficient and sleep-deprived groups, it is revealed that doing homework as the last activity before bedtime is much more likely to occur in the sleep-deprived group than in the sleep-sufficient group, especially among adolescents aged 12–14 and 15–17 years old. This phenomenon is particularly prominent among adolescents aged 12–14 and 15–17.

Table 8.11 Main pre-bedtime activities of children and adolescents (including naps) Unit: %

Age	Activity	The proportion of the sleep-deprived	The proportion of the sleep-sufficient
6–11	Doing homework	16.7	12.0
	Watching TV	42.1	40.2
	Playing computer games	2.6	1.4
12–14	Doing homework	38.8	18.1
	Watching TV	16.1	34.1
	Playing computer games	2.4	2.7
15–17	Doing homework	34.2	20.2
	Watching TV	2.3	17.3
	Playing computer games	4.6	6.9

Table 8.12 Main pre-bedtime activities of children and adolescents (excluding naps) Unit: %

Age	Activity	The proportion of the sleep-deprived	The proportion of the sleep-sufficient
6–11	Doing homework	16.3	10.0
	Watching TV	42.2	38.5
	Playing computer games	2.4	1.1
12–14	Doing homework	32.1	15.3
	Watching TV	18.1	39.4
	Playing computer games	2.4	2.8
15–17	Doing homework	35.7	14.0
	Watching TV	4.8	21.0
	Playing computer games	3.0	8.9

Next, we further analyzed the time use of doing homework, watching TV, and playing computer games during the day for both sleep-deprived and sleep-sufficient children. Tables 8.13 and 8.14 record the main time use of the sleep-deprived group and the sleep-sufficient group. The statistical results show that the sleep-deprived group spent more time doing homework than the sleep-sufficient, and in terms of mean values, the sleep-deprived group spent nearly twice as much time doing homework as the sleep-sufficient group among adolescents aged 15–17 (see Table 8.14), further demonstrating that long homework time is the primary cause of sleep deprivation among children and adolescents.

This suggests that time spent doing homework and self-perceived academic stress may all be strongly associated with sleep duration, latency, and quality in the more senior grades. Among older students, the time spent doing homework not only affects the total time spent sleeping, but also relates to the quality of sleep. In contrast, among younger students, self-perceived academic stress rather than time spent doing homework impacted sleep quality. Such results are a unique phenomenon in Asian countries, reflecting the importance that Asian families place on the academic achievement of children and adolescents, and also reminding us to keep homework time within reasonable limits and to reduce students' academic stress appropriately.

Table 8.13 Average length of doing homework, watching tv and playing computer games (including naps) among children and adolescents Unit: hours/day

Age	Activity	The proportion of the sleep-deprived					The proportion of the sleep-sufficient				
		Mean value	Urban		Rural		Mean Value	Urban		Rural	
			Male	Female	Male	Female		Male	Female	Male	Female
6–11	Doing homework	1.46	2.61	1.51	1.99	1.24	1.27	1.25	1.41	0.88	0.81
	Watching TV	1.62	1.02	0.90	1.22	1.04	1.52	1.38	1.26	1.88	1.66
	Playing computer games	0.24	0.31	0.84	–	–	0.12	0.21	0.06	0.10	0.04
12–14	Doing homework	2.08	2.34	2.54	1.47	1.83	1.57	1.60	2.12	1.04	1.46
	Watching TV	0.74	0.35	0.30	1.14	0.71	1.50	1.56	0.08	1.36	2.08
	Playing computer games	0.25	0.31	0.84	–	–	0.21	0.20	0.03	0.40	0.19
15–17	Doing homework	2.17	2.13	2.60	1.39	2.63	1.34	1.55	1.74	0.72	1.23
	Watching TV	0.21	0.26	0.08	0.31	0.10	1.13	0.87	1.24	1.19	1.28
	Playing computer games	0.12	0.26	0.01	0.05	–	0.70	0.98	0.41	1.09	0.14

Table 8.14 Average length of doing homework, watching tv and playing computer games for children and adolescents (excluding naps) Unit: hours/day

Age	Activity	The proportion of the sleep-deprived					The proportion of the sleep-sufficient				
		Mean value	Urban		Rural		Mean Value	Urban		Rural	
			Male	Female	Male	Female		Male	Female	Male	Female
6–11	Doing homework	1.43	1.72	1.69	1.2	1.22	0.99	1.13	1.36	0.70	0.77
	Watching TV	1.44	1.50	1.13	1.74	1.28	1.69	1.55	1.41	1.93	1.69
	Playing computer games	0.18	0.22	0.16	0.19	0.11	0.13	0.24	0.06	0.14	0.01
12–14	Doing homework	1.78	1.85	2.28	1.24	1.67	1.60	1.69	2.25	1.02	1.41
	Watching TV	0.73	0.68	0.47	1.02	0.94	1.79	1.88	1.24	1.58	2.57
	Playing computer games	0.15	0.12	0.02	0.15	0.04	0.28	0.26	0.05	0.56	0.27
15–17	Doing homework	2.09	2.50	2.57	1.22	2.08	1.10	1.28	1.51	0.79	1.11
	Watching TV	0.36	0.10	0.17	0.36	0.71	1.35	1.15	1.54	1.26	1.24
	Playing computer games	0.18	0.28	0.03	0.31	0.02	0.86	1.26	0.39	1.14	0.21

Among elementary school students, there was a negative correlation between the time spent playing video games and the length of sleep. This finding is consistent with the study by Yogesh et al.[15] Children and adolescents have insufficient control over the time spent on cell phones and have problems in trying to reduce the time spent on cell phones, which leads to a prolongation of cell phone use and consequently a reduction in sleep duration. Some even show a stronger desire to use their phones when they are not around and have problems such as repeatedly checking their phones, which affects sleep duration.

Notably, the structure of time use changed very significantly among sleep-deprived elementary, junior high, and senior high school students. TV viewing time was negatively correlated with age, with a significant decrease in TV viewing time with increasing age. A possible explanation is that older students are affected by academic pressure and watch significantly less TV time.

A regression analysis based on a discrete choice model was needed to identify further the factors influencing sleep among children and adolescents. We assigned a value of 1 to sleep deprivation and 0 to sleep adequacy, and conducted a logit

[15] Yogesh S., Abha S., Pariyanka S., "Mobile Usage and Sleep Patterns among Medical Students", *Physical Pharmacol*, 2014, 58 (1).

Table 8.15 Analysis of sleep influencing factors

	Sufficiency of sleep		
	6–11	12–14	15–17
Mother's education level	−0.014	0.107	0.252**
	(0.061)	(0.093)	(0.099)
Grades	0.061	0.134	−0.224**
	(0.066)	(0.103)	(0.112)
Time spent doing homework before bed	0.394***	0.409***	0.323***
	(0.078)	(0.078)	(0.077)
Family income level	0.067	0.013	0.083
	(0.098)	(0.141)	(0.152)
Is the father home (0 = yes; 1 = no)	0.413	0.126	0.264
	(0.324)	(0.387)	(0.521)
Gender (0 = female; 1 = male)	0.038	−0.063	0.109
	(0.108)	(0.160)	(0.176)
Urban–rural division (0 = urban; 1 = rural)	0.266**	0.004	−0.110
	(0.120)	(0.176)	(0.200)
Constant term	−0.141	−1.098**	−0.803*
	(0.286)	(0.442)	(0.447)
Observed value	1491	715	593

Note Standard errors are in parentheses, and ***, **, and * indicate that the estimated coefficients passed significance tests at the 1, 5, and 10% levels, respectively

regression. The regression results in Table 8.15 show that[16] homework time before bedtime significantly affects children and adolescents' sleep, controlling for urban–rural, income, and parental companionship factors. If other factors are held constant, each one-hour increase in homework time before bedtime will increase the probability of sleep deprivation by about 39.4% for students aged 6–11, by about 40.9% for students aged 12–14, and by about 32.3% for students aged 15–17.

Summary

This chapter analyzed the sleep problems of Chinese children and adolescents using data from the 2017 Chinese Time Use Survey. The analysis shows that nationally, when naptime is included, children and adolescents aged 6–11 years sleep an average of 10.67 h per day, children and adolescents aged 12–14 years sleep an average of

[16] We found that the regression results of the significance and the direction of influence of the influencing factors were consistent whether nap time was included or not, so here we only report the regression results without nap time.

9.85 h per day, and children and adolescents aged 15–17 years sleep an average of 9.25 h per day, and the sleep deprivation rates of children and adolescents in the three age groups were 31.0, 22.2 and 20.2% respectively.

If nap time is not included, the average sleep duration for children and adolescents aged 6–11 years in China is 9.79 h per day, with 9.00 h per day for children and adolescents aged 12–14 years, and 8.29 h per day for children and adolescents aged 15–17 years. The sleep deprivation rate among children and adolescents remains high, with 54.7, 43.7 and 41.7% for the three age groups, respectively. Children aged 6–11 and 12–14 whose academic performance was above average or below were most likely to be sleep-deprived, while high achiever children ages 15–17 were most likely to be sleep-deprived.

From an international comparative perspective, the sleep duration of Chinese children and adolescents is significantly lower compared to developed countries such as the United States; from a comparative analysis across time, the sleep deprivation rate of children and adolescents decreased significantly in 2017 compared to 2012, and the sleep situation improved. In particular, it should be noted that the main factor leading to sleep deprivation among Chinese children and adolescents is the long time spent on homework.

The above analysis may give us the following insights. First, the groups of children and adolescents who are most likely to suffer from sleep deprivation are those with upper-middle academic performance and below, and those who spend more time on homework, which means that reducing the burden of students is still the right topic; second, from the perspective of children and adolescents' growth, the poor academic performance, long homework time and sleep deprivation may form a vicious circle: poor academic performance requires intensive study and more homework, which in turn leads to insufficient sleep, and insufficient sleep further affects academic performance.

Chapter 9
"Happy" College Students

"The children are desperately studying when they should be playing; the young people are desperately playing games when they should be studying." On June 21st, 2018, Minister of Education Chen Baosheng said at the National Conference on Undergraduate Education in the New Era that the phenomenon of "hard-working high schools and happy universities" in Chinese education should be reversed, and that "the burden should be effectively reduced for primary and middle school students and reasonably increased for college students", so as to enhance the raise challenges of college students.[1] Compared with the busy high school life, after entering university, the time and form of classes have been greatly adjusted, and students have the right to choose between study and leisure to a large extent, so they have significantly more time at their disposal. College students are mainly self-management; how to make good use of study time efficiently and how to make good use of after-school time are important questions that contemporary college students need to think deeply about.[2]

According to a study, only 12.3% of college students spend more than 8 h in class every day on average, and with the change in class format, half of the students can concentrate on listening for 30–40 min in each class (50 min a lesson for example); the main reason that affects listening to class is playing with cell phones.[3] University students' after-school time use is rooted in the campus life culture.[4] Making full use of after-school time and arranging after-school life reasonably are important guidelines for college students' professional quality and career planning. Research

[1] News from the Central People's Government of the People's Republic of China, http://www.gov.cn/xinwen/2018-06/21/content_5300316.htm.

[2] Feixia Hu, "Investigation and Analysis on the Utilization of College Students' After-school Time—Taking Anhui University as an Example", *Social Survey*, 2017 (8).

[3] Yan Cui, "Research on College Students' Study Time and Coping Strategies—Taiyuan University of Technology as an Example", *Education Teaching Forum*, 2018 (10).

[4] Qiang Li, "Analysis of the Influencing Factors of College Students' After-School Time Utilization—A Questionnaire Survey Based on Tianjin Haihe Education Park", *Journal of Capital University of Economics and Business*, 2014 (6).

F. Du et al., *Chinese People's Time Use and Their Quality of Life*,
https://doi.org/10.1007/978-981-99-5526-8_9

shows that many college students' after-school time utilization has problems such as low efficiency, lack of planning, and high negative impact of after-school life.[5]

Using data from the 2017 Chinese Time Use Survey, this chapter explores college students' time use in activities such as studying, sleeping, recreation, and reading based on comparative analysis, and compares it with high school students and finally with American college students' time use. The analysis found that compared to high school students, college students spent significantly less time studying, more time sleeping, more time recreating, and more time reading on electronic devices; compared to US college students, Chinese college students spent more time in classes and sleeping and less time on extracurricular learning and leisure socializing.

The analysis in this chapter is based on a sample of high school and college students from the 2017 Chinese Time Use Survey. The total sample size was 885, including 487 high school students and 398 college students. To analyze the differences within the college student group, the sample was divided into college students (135) and undergraduates (263).

Considering the characteristics of the activities that students engage in, this chapter divides students' activities in a day into four major categories: self-care, study, leisure and social, and other activities. The specific classifications are shown in Table 9.1.

The activities that students engage in can be further divided into two categories: non-discretionary activities and discretionary activities, depending on the flexibility of each type of activity. Classes are scheduled by the school, and students are not free to choose the length and starting and ending times of these activities. All activities other than classes are discretionary, and students are more or less free to consider their time schedule.

Stage Features of Students' Time Use

In order to examine the characteristics of students' time allocation at different educational stages, this section compares the time use of students[6] at each stage (elementary school, junior high school, senior high school, and university), as shown in Fig. 9.1.

As shown in Fig. 9.1, the college level is a departure from the trend from elementary to high school in terms of study time, self-care, and leisure and social time. From elementary school to high school, the average time spent studying goes up, cumulatively rising by 2.15 h per day, reflecting a continuous increase in study pressure; after college, the time spent studying drops dramatically by 3.60 h per day, reflecting a steep decline in study pressure. From elementary school to high school, the average time spent on self-care and leisure and social activities went downward,

[5] Haining Zhao, Feng Zhu, "Analysis of the Influence of College Students' After-School Time-use Status on Professional Quality—A Survey Based on Students from the School of Management, Xinjiang Agricultural University", *Human Resource Management*, 2018 (1).

[6] Sample sizes of students at each stage: 1,782 elementary school students, 731 junior school students, 487 senior high school students, and 398 college students.

Table 9.1 Classification of students' activities

Category	Activities included	Activity description	Flexibility
Studying	Attending classes	Students engage in school-organized learning activities at school	Non-discretionary
	Learning outside of class	Writing assignments, pre-reading, research, and other learning activities	Discretionary
Self-care	Sleeping at night	Prolonged sleep to meet physiological needs	
	Other sleep	Sleep activities other than those listed above	
	Personal hygiene	Daily personal hygiene activities for oneself	
	Eating	Activities of ingesting various foods and drinks	
Leisure and social activities	Playing games	Cell phone games and computer games	
	Physical exercise	Physical activities for health promotion and mental regulation by using various physical means according to physical needs	
	Social interaction	Various forms of social interaction with friends, relatives or others	
	Amateur hobbies	Singing, collecting, literature, art, etc.	
	Watching TV	Watching TV	
	Reading	Reading e-books and reading paperback books	
Other activities	Paid labor	Work and home production activities	
	Unpaid labor	Housework, caring for family members and offering external help	

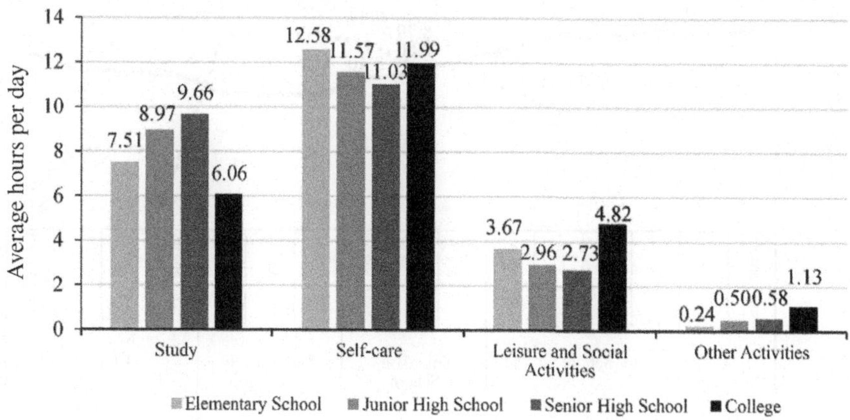

Fig. 9.1 Time allocation of students at different learning stages. *Source* 2017 Chinese Time Use Survey, the same below

with the former dropping by 1.55 h per day and the latter by 0.94 h per day; after college, the time spent on self-care and leisure and social activities both increased significantly, with the former rising by 0.96 h per day and the latter by 2.09 h per day. As for other activities, there was a small increase from elementary school to high school, and the increase climbed significantly after going to university. Comparing students at all stages, college students had the shortest study time, the longest leisure and social time, and the most comfortable life.

Figure 9.2 shows the average amount of time spent studying and sleeping at night for students at each grade level at different stages of study. It is obvious that from first grade in elementary school to the third grade in senior high school, study time and Nighttime sleep duration are scissors-shaped: study time gradually increased and Nighttime sleep duration gradually decreased; the two intersected between the first and second grades, before which nighttime sleep was higher than study time, and after which study time was longer than sleep time; the increase of study time reflects the rise of study pressure; the decline in nighttime sleep reflects a decline in the amount of sleep people biologically need as they get older, as well as a shift away from sleep by studying. After going to university, this trend was broken: study time fell off a cliff and nighttime sleep rose against physiological needs.

Figure 9.3 shows students' average time spent on reading, playing games, and physical exercise by different study levels by grade. It can be seen that students' time spent reading, playing games, and physical exercise was generally on the rise from the first grade of elementary school to the third grade of senior high school, dropping back at high school, and rising sharply by the freshman year.

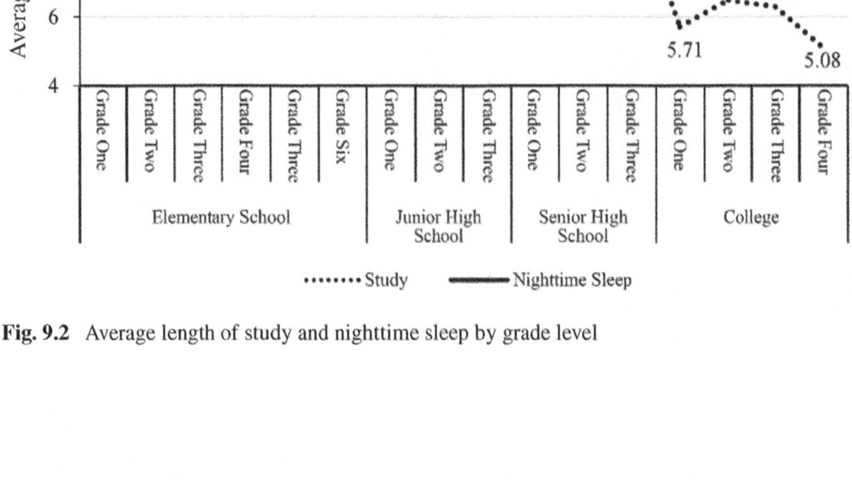

Fig. 9.2 Average length of study and nighttime sleep by grade level

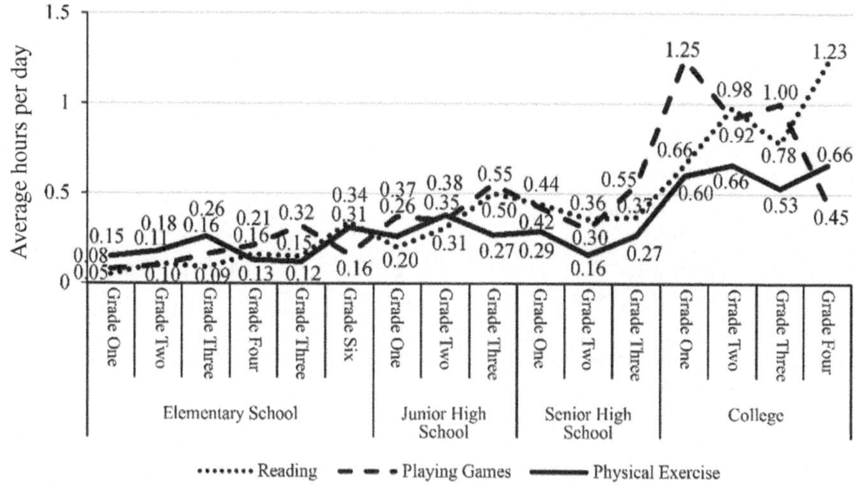

Fig. 9.3 Average length of reading, playing games, and physical exercise for students by grades

Comparison of Time Use Between College Students and Senior High School Students

This section compares the time use of college students and high school students in four major categories of activities, as well as the differences between junior college students and undergraduates, as shown in Table 9.2 and Fig. 9.4.

As shown in Table 9.2 and Fig. 9.4, students' study intensity decreased significantly after college. Compared with high school students, college students' study time decreased by 3.60 h/day, or as much as 37%; among them, college students' study time fell especially sharply, or as much as 44%. The participation rate of college students in learning activities also dropped significantly by about 10% points compared with that of high school students.

In contrast to the direction of change in academic activities, students spent significantly more time on self-care, leisure and socialization, and other activities after college. Compared with high school students, college students spent 0.96 h/day more on self-care, an increase of 9%; 2.09 h per day more on leisure and social activities, an increase of 77%, with 91% for junior college students; and 0.55 h per day more on other activities, an increase of 95%.

It can be seen that, compared with senior high school students, the overall characteristics of time allocation of college students are that the time spent on studying is significantly reduced and the time spent on other activities such as leisure and social activities is significantly increased. This is analyzed in detail in the next four sections of this chapter.

Table 9.2 Overall time use of high school and college students

Activity	Indicator	Senior high school students	Total college students	#Junior college students	#Undergraduates
Study	Average hours per day	9.66	6.06	5.42	6.33
	Participation rate (%)	83.1	73.2	73.3	73.2
	Participant length (hours/day)	11.63	8.27	7.40	8.65
Self-care	Average hours per day	11.03	11.99	12.08	11.96
	Participation rate (%)	100.0	100.0	100.0	100.0
	Participant length (hours/day)	11.03	11.99	12.08	11.96
Leisure and social activities	Average hours per day	2.73	4.82	5.21	4.65
	Participation rate (%)	66.3	91.7	94.0	90.7
	Participant length (hours/day)	4.11	5.25	5.55	5.12
Other activities	Average hours per day	0.58	1.13	1.28	1.07
	Participation rate (%)	19.4	30.7	36.2	28.3
	Participant length (hours/day)	2.98	3.69	3.54	3.77

Significant Decrease in Studying Time

This section compares the time use of college and high school students in terms of study, as well as the differences between college specialists and undergraduates. The basic picture of which is shown in Fig. 9.5.

As shown in Fig. 9.5, college students spent much less time in class than high school students. Compared with high school students, undergraduates spent 2.79 h per day less in class, a decrease of 37%, while college students spent 3.04 h per day less in class, a decrease of 40%. There was also a significant reduction in time spent studying outside of class after college, by about 1/4 for undergraduates and more than half for specialists.

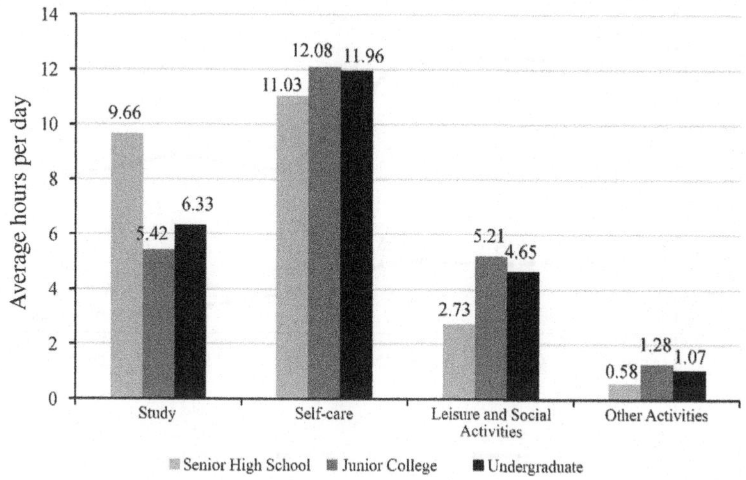

Fig. 9.4 Time allocation of high school and college students

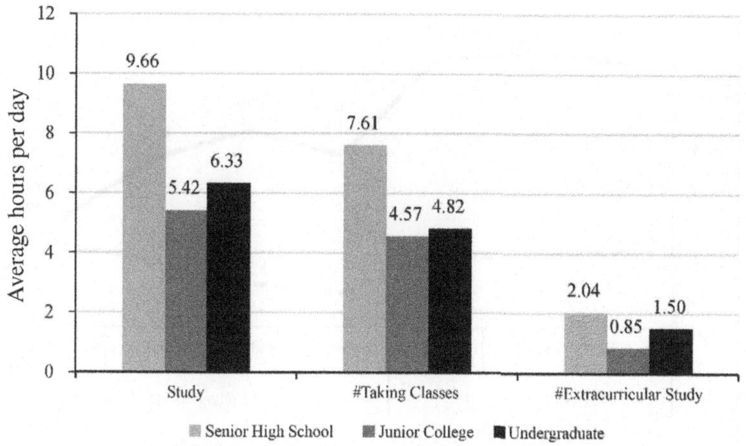

Fig. 9.5 Distribution of study time between senior high school and junior college students

Figures 9.6 and 9.7 show the changes of classroom and extracurricular studying time by grades.

As seen in Figs. 9.6 and 9.7, there is a significant jump in the amount of time students spend in class and extracurricular study from their senior year to their freshman year. Class time for senior high school students remained above 7.5 h per day for all grades, with little difference. After moving to freshman year, class time jumped to 4.5–4.9 h per day, a decrease of about 40%. Class time for college students increased slightly from freshman to sophomore year and decreased slightly by junior year; by senior year for undergraduates, class time decreased again significantly. For

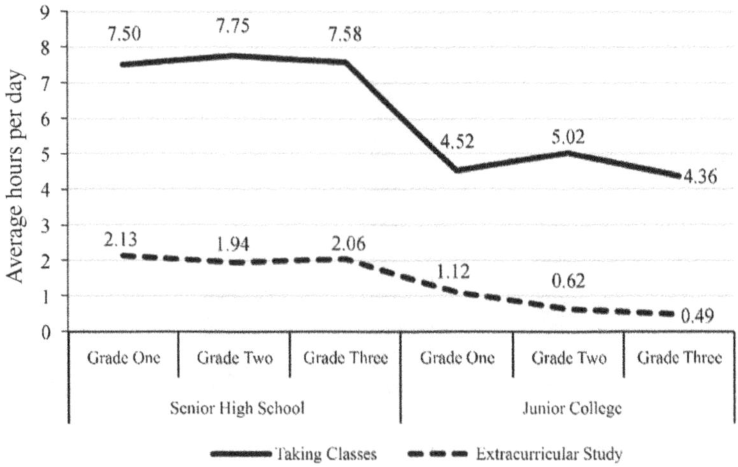

Fig. 9.6 Class and extracurricular study time for high school and college students by grade level

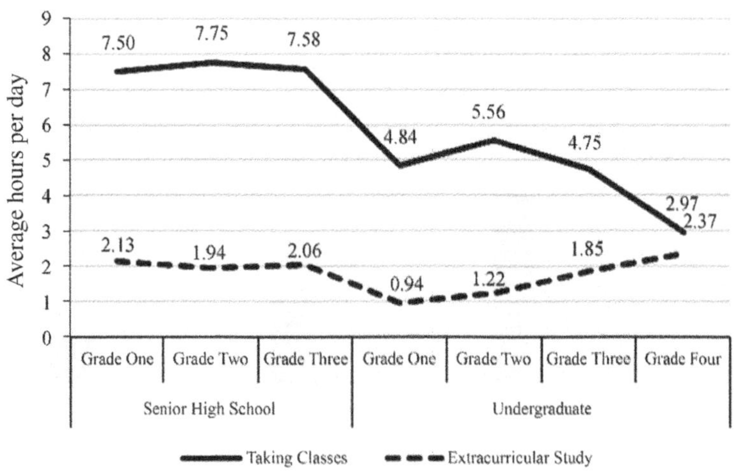

Fig. 9.7 Time spent in and out of class for senior high school and college undergraduates by grades

students, class time is not discretionary; the jump and drop in class time from high school to college, as well as the change in class time between college years, primarily reflect differences in teaching schedules at each level. Course pressure is much lower in college than in high school, and again much lower in the senior-high year than in freshman through junior year in college.

There are differences and similarities in the extracurricular study time and class. High school students spend about 2 h a day studying outside of class at each grade level, with little variation between grades. After entering freshman year, class time jumped to about 1 h per day, a drop of up to 50%. The amount of time spent studying outside of class for college students went all the way down from freshman to junior year for specialists and increased significantly from freshman to senior year for undergraduates. For students, extracurricular study time was largely at their disposal; the jump and drop in extracurricular study time from high school to college, as well as the change in extracurricular study time between college years, mainly reflect the differences in students' learning initiatives at each stage. Due to the great pressure of the college entrance examination, high school students still devoted a lot of time to completing homework and pre-studying and reviewing their homework on top of the heavy class load. Compared with high school, college education is characterized by significantly fewer class hours, but requires students to complete a great deal of reading, research, and other tasks outside of class. Because of the generally low academic demands placed on students in college, this assumption falls flat: college students do not devote the reduced class time to study outside of class.

In response to the general laxity of university students' studies, on August 27th, 2018, the Ministry of Education issued a *Notice on the Implementation of the Spirit of the National Conference on Undergraduate Education in the New Era*, which called for "a comprehensive overhaul of the education and teaching order, strict management of the teaching process of undergraduate education, enhancing the management of the learning process, and urge universities to comprehensively sort out the teaching content of each course, eliminating 'easy-A classes', creating 'golden courses', reasonably enhancing the academic challenge, increasing the difficulty of the courses, expanding the depth of the courses, and effectively improving the teaching quality of the courses. Strengthen the assessment of the learning process, increase the proportion of the process assessment results in the total grade of the course, and resolutely abolish the final exam system that aims at approving students to pass so that they can graduate.[7]" Raising the academic requirements is conducive to college students making good use of their more flexible time and improving their time management skills so that they can be more competitive in the future job market. In addition, while paying attention to the study of university undergraduates, the study of junior college students is equally noteworthy.

Significant Increase in Sleep Time

A large portion of the reduced study time is spent on sleep by college students, as shown in Fig. 9.8.

As shown in Fig. 9.8, compared to high school students, college students' nighttime sleep increased significantly; undergraduates increased by 0.57 h per day, or 7%, and specialists increased by 0.94 h per day, or 12%. There was also a small increase in nap and eating time after going to college.

Figures 9.9 and 9.10 show the change in nighttime sleep duration by grade.

---

[7] Ministry of Education of the People's Republic of China, http://www.moe.gov.cn/srcsite/A08/s7056/201809/t20180903_347079.html?from=timeline&isappinstalled=0.

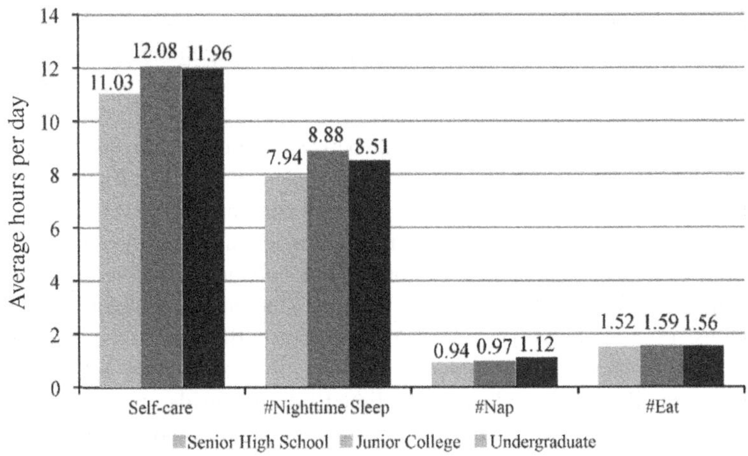

Fig. 9.8 Time allocation of self-care for senior high school and college students

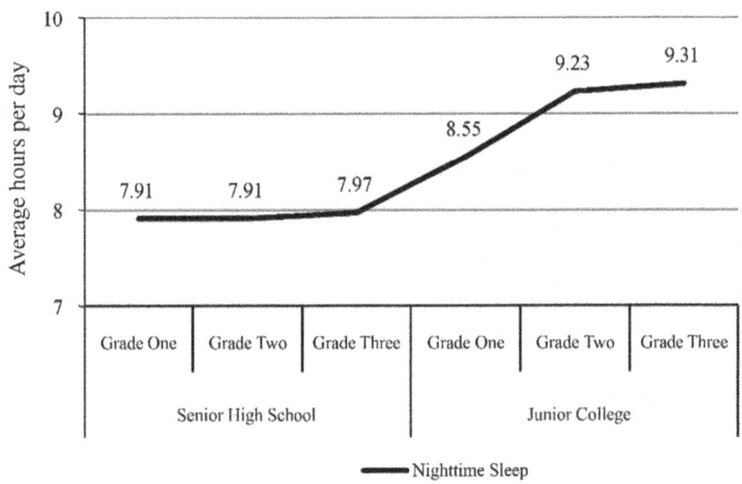

Fig. 9.9 Nighttime sleep duration of high school and college students by grade

As shown in Figs. 9.9 and 9.10, there was a significant increase in nighttime sleep duration for students after attending college. Nighttime sleep duration for high school students remained close to 8 h per day, with little difference between grade levels. For college specialists, nighttime sleep duration rose two levels in a row from senior to freshman year and freshman to sophomore year, finally exceeding 9.2 h per day. For undergraduates, nighttime sleep duration reached 8.4 h per day from senior year to freshman to junior year; by senior year, it further increased to about 9.1 h per day.

The free time available to college students, excluding the fixed time for classes, increased dramatically. Due to the lack of proper time planning, some college students

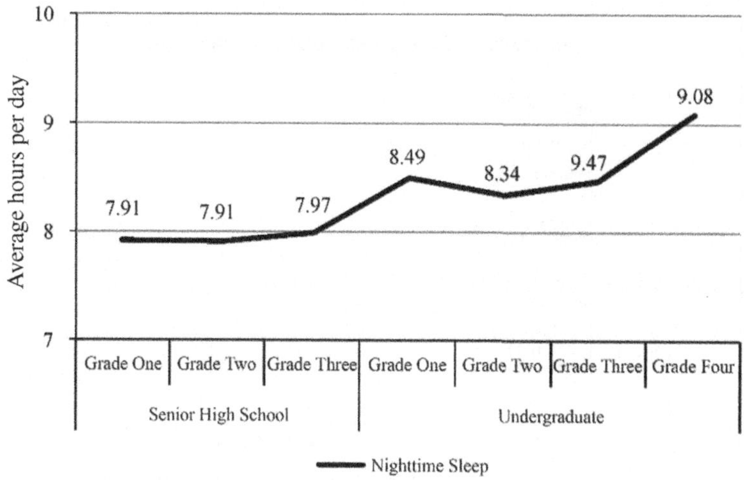

Fig. 9.10 Nighttime sleep duration of high school and college undergraduates by grade

sleep in the dormitory to kill time. They attend classes on time and sleep at other times. They are called the "sleepers".

Significant Increase in Recreational Time

Some of the time released by studying after going to college is used for sleeping, but a larger portion is used by students for leisure and recreation, especially playing games.

The vigorous development and widespread use of Internet technology has greatly changed people's way of communication, thinking patterns and behavior patterns. The obsession of college students with the Internet is undeniable; some have even reached the level of addiction.[8] According to a university's data, "the number of Internet users in the dormitory exceeds 34,000, accounting for about 92% of the students in the university".[9] Incidents of academic neglect, emotional outbursts, and behavioral disorders caused by college students' indulgence in online games are constantly appearing. The destructive nature of online game addiction has become a hot issue of concern for the government, society and universities.[10] In the new edition of the *International Classification of Diseases* released by the World Health

[8] Wenjin Fu, Xinxin Chen, "An Analysis of College Students' Internet Addiction", Ability and Wisdom, 2017 (17).

[9] Weijun Zhang, Jiaping Zhu, Weizang Bian, Yuliang Wang, "Survey and Analysis of College Students' After-School Time-use", *Guide to Business*, 2012 (5).

[10] Guangming Huang, Lijuan An, "The Causes and Countermeasures of Online Game Addiction Among College Students," *Modern Business Trade Industry*, 2017 (18).

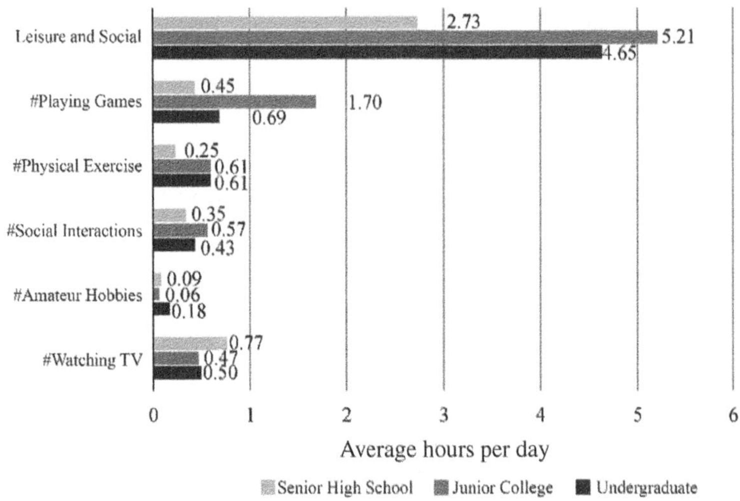

Fig. 9.11 Allocation of leisure and social time of senior high school and college students

Organization in 2018, gaming disorder (commonly known as gaming addiction) was added to the chapter on addictive disease. Game addiction has attracted a high level of attention. In this section, we analyze the allocation of leisure time among college students by comparing it with high school students. The basic situation in this regard is shown in Fig. 9.11.

As seen in Fig. 9.11, compared with high school students, the leisure social time of college students increased significantly. After going to university, the playing time of undergraduates increased by 0.24 h per day, an increase of more than 50%; the playing time of junior college students increased by 1.25 h per day, an alarming increase of 178%. The physical exercise time of college students has increased by 0.36 h per day, an increment of 144%. The social interaction time of college students also increased significantly. The amateur hobby time of undergraduates increased while that of junior college students decreased, and the time of watching TV decreased significantly.

Figures 9.12 and 9.13 show the changes in playing games and physical exercise time by grade.

As shown in Figs. 9.12 and 9.13, after going to college, college students, especially junior college students, spent significantly more time playing games and considerably more time on physical exercise. The playing time of senior high school students was more restrained, about 0.4 h per day in each grade. From senior year in high school to freshman year, the playing time of college students soared 2.4 times, and fell back in sophomore and junior years; the increase of playing time of undergraduates was much smaller. The apparent increase in college students' playing time is probably because electronic devices such as cell phones and computers have become essential items for contemporary college students. When they first enter university, the learning mode turns to independent learning. Without the pressure of heavy coursework and

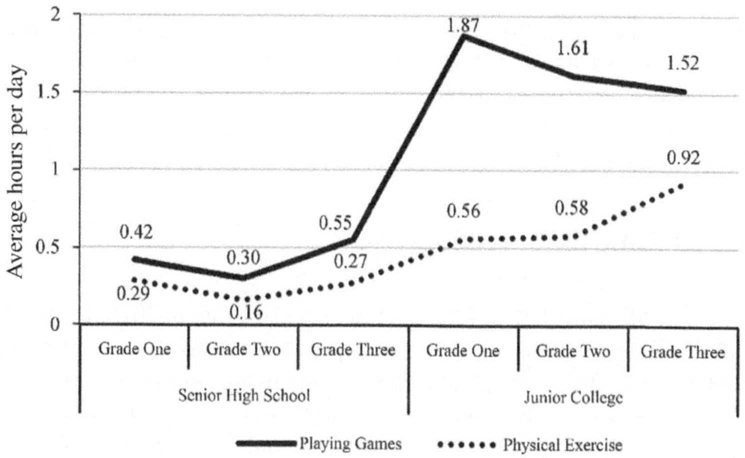

Fig. 9.12 Time spent playing games and physical exercise by grades for high school students and junior college students

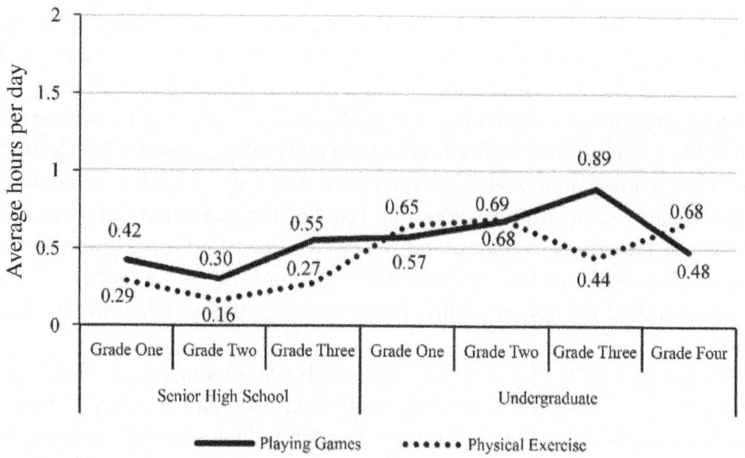

Fig. 9.13 Time spent playing games and physical activity by grades for high school and undergraduates

supervision of parents and teachers, the temptation of online games makes newly enrolled college students spend more time playing games.

The exercise time of senior high school students in each grade is maintained at about 0.25 h per day. From senior year in high school to freshman year, the exercise time of college students increased significantly by 1.1 times. Subsequently, the exercise time of junior college students continued to increase, and that of undergraduates fluctuated slightly.

Under test-based education, high school students' study and life focus on college entrance exams, and study squeezes out recreation time. After the college entrance exams, students seem to lose their direction, and without the pressure of exams, college becomes a paradise for recreation and leisure.

Increased Time for E-reading

The results of the *13th National Reading Survey* show that in 2015, Chinese adults read 7.86 books per capita, including 4.58 paperback books and 3.21 e-books; in recent years, China has seen a slight improvement in the number of books read, and a greater rise in reading time in emerging media, with significant growth in cell phone reading. The US *Reading Report 2016* shows that adults in the US read 12 books in 2015, with more paperback books than e-books and audio books. It can be seen that compared with the United States, reading time in China is significantly lower.[11] The education level of Chinese people is significantly lower than that of the United States, which may explain why Chinese people read less than the United States.[12] According to the *Human Development Report 2016* released by the United Nations, the average number of years of education in China in 2015 was 7.6 years, while the average number of years of education in the United States was 13.2 years.

Students are a major part of the reading population. Figure 9.14 show the distribution of reading time among senior high school and college students. It is important to note that the reading analyzed in the later part of this section refers to reading other than academics. Some studies show that reading for recreation purposes accounts for 87.3% of paperback reading, and 81.2% of electronic reading among college students.[13] Reading outside of academics accounts for the majority of reading. Therefore, reading for non-academic purposes can roughly reflect the total reading situation.

As shown in Fig. 9.14, compared with high school students, college students' reading time has increased, including 0.49 h/day for junior college students, an increase of 1.3 times, and 0.46 h per day for undergraduates, an increase of 1.2 times. The increase in reading time mainly occurred in electronic reading, and the time spent on paperbacks did not change much. Regarding the proportion of paperback reading time to total reading time, the proportion of paperback reading time was 31% for high

[11] Zhiping Xia, "Analysis and Implications of the Latest National Reading Survey Report in China and the United States", *Library Research*, 2017 (5).

[12] There is evidence that the higher the education level, the more reading is done. According to data from the 2017 China Time-use Survey, for residents aged 18 and older, reading time increases as education increases. The average time spent reading when the education levels are unschooled, elementary school, junior high school, senior high school, technical secondary school or secondary vocational school, junior college or vocational high school, and university undergraduate and above are 0.02 h/day, 0.11 h/day, 0.25 h/day, 0.38 h/day, 0.45 h/day, 0.54 h/day, and 0.66 h/day, respectively.

[13] Jiao Qu, Jing Bai, Ning Wang, "An Empirical Study of College Students' Book Reading Behavior", *Journal of Academic Library and Information Science*, 2017 (5).

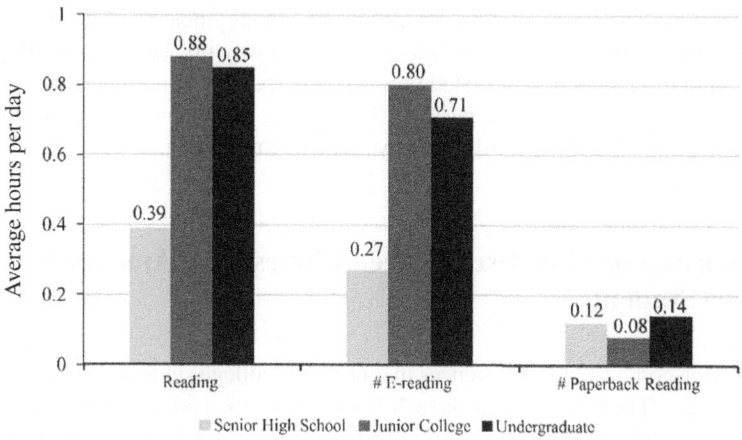

Fig. 9.14 Reading time allocation of senior high school and college students

school students, 16% for university undergraduates, and 9% for college students. It can be seen that the proportion of paperback reading among college students decreased significantly.

Figure 9.15 shows the e-reading and paperback reading time changes by grade.

As shown in Fig. 9.15, the amount of time spent e-reading by high school students decreases slightly as the grade level increases. From senior year in high school to

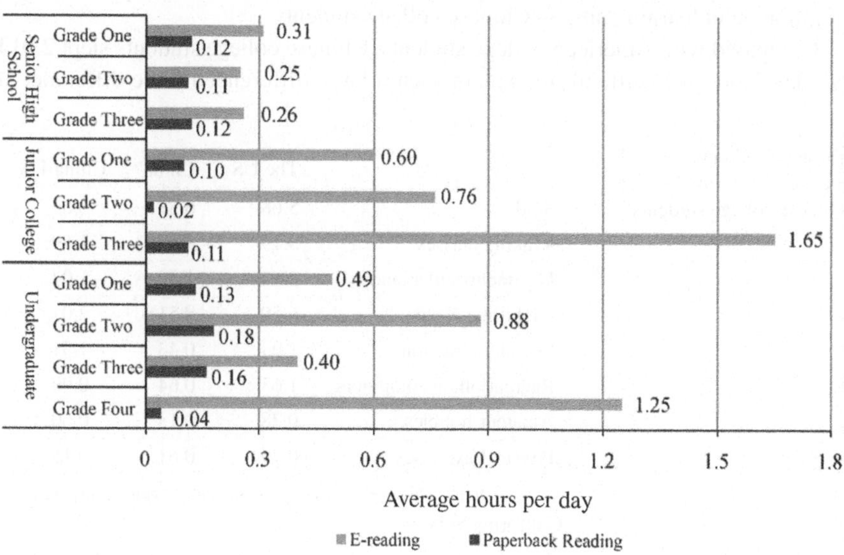

Fig. 9.15 E-reading and paperback reading time of high school students, junior college students and undergraduates by grade

freshman year, the time spent on e-reading jumped significantly. After that, the e-reading time of junior college students went all the way up, and the e-reading time of undergraduate students oscillated upward. Paperback reading time was generally low, averaging less than 0.2 h per day. Apparently, the time released by studying after going to university is partly used by students for reading.

Comparison of Time Use Between Chinese and American College Students

This section compares the differences in time use of college students in China and the United States. The US data are from a 2006 survey by the University of California,[14] which was conducted among undergraduate students. The Chinese data are from a sample of undergraduate students in the 2017 Chinese Time Use Survey. There are some differences in how these two surveys were interviewed, but they are roughly comparable in terms of classifying college students' activities. The comparative results are shown in Table 9.3.

As shown in Table 9.3, compared with American college students, Chinese college students spent 0.65 h per day more time studying, including 1.69 h per day more time in class and 1.04 h per day less time studying outside of class. The difference in class time reflects the difference in class schedules between the two countries, with Chinese universities having a higher number of class hours. Notably, Chinese college students have much lower extracurricular study time, which reflects a significant lack of initiative in learning among Chinese college students.

Compared with American college students, Chinese college students slept 2.01 h per day more. It is difficult to explain such a large difference by the difference in

Table 9.3 Comparison of time use between US and Chinese college students. Unit: hours/day

	The US	China	China-US
Study	5.68	6.33	0.65
#Taking classes	3.13	4.82	1.69
#Extracurricular study	2.54	1.50	−1.04
Nighttime sleep	6.50	8.51	2.01
Social interactions	1.94	0.43	−1.51
Recreation on computers	1.63	0.64	−0.99
Amateur hobbies	0.78	0.18	−0.60
Physical exercise	0.79	0.61	−0.18

Source 2017 Chinese Time Use Survey, 2006 University of California Survey

[14] Brint S., Cantwell A. M., "Undergraduate Time Use and Academic Outcomes: Results from the University of California Undergraduate Experience Survey 2006", *Teachers College Record*, 2010, 112 (9).

access patterns. The fact that Chinese college students spent more time on sleep may be due to the fact that Chinese universities were not rich enough in after-school life to draw students away from their enthusiasm for sleep. Indeed, Chinese college students spent less time on social interaction, using computers for recreation, hobbies, and physical activity than American college students.

Summary

This chapter explores the time allocation of Chinese college students and compares it with that of senior high school students, and finally compares it with the time use of American college students. The major findings are as follows.

Compared with high school students, college students' study and life are much easier: class time is reduced by about 40%, and there is a substantial reduction in extracurricular study time. Part of the time released by studying is used by students for sleeping and reading, and a larger part is used by students for leisure and recreation, especially playing games.

Among college students, junior college students have easier lives than undergraduates: the former spend less time in class and studying outside of class, and more time playing games and sleeping at night.

Compared with American college students, Chinese college students spend more time in class and less time studying outside of class. This reflects a significant lack of initiative in learning among Chinese college students. Chinese college students sleep more and spend less time on leisure and social life. This reflects that Chinese college students' after-school life needs to be richer.

From the analysis of this chapter, we can get the following insights. First, reforming the existing education system, effectively reducing the burden of primary and secondary school students and increasing the burden of college students are urgent tasks for cultivating college students. Second, the focus of increasing the burden of college students does not lie in increasing the class hours, but in raising the academic requirements, prompting college students to increase the time for extracurricular study such as homework, reading and research, and enhancing their independent learning ability. The era of a knowledge-driven economy requires college students to have the ability of continuous learning in order not to be eliminated by the times. Third, college students have more discretionary time, and it is essential to cultivate students' time management ability. Life is made up of time. College students should learn to plan their time reasonably and improve their efficiency of time use, which will not only fulfill and enrich their study and life during college, but also benefit them for a lifetime.

Part IV
After Work: The Pursuit of Quality of Life

Chapter 10
Social Difference in Leisure and Social Activities

Leisure and social activities refer to the activities people engage in their free time after completing paid labor, unpaid labor, studying and training, and self-care, which includes sports and fitness, reading, hobbies, watching TV, resting, socializing, etc. Leisure and social activities reflect people's allocation and use of free time. These activities help to improve physical and mental health, establish, maintain and expand social circles, and are an important investment in human capital and social capital. More importantly, leisure and social activities are the main sources of satisfaction. Therefore, the quantity and quality of leisure and social activities can be used to measure residents' quality of life directly.

Like other consumption activities, leisure and social activities also require a certain amount of time and material investment. Since different social groups have diversified discretionary time and material investment, and their preferences for various types of leisure and social activities vary widely, they diverge significantly among different social groups.[1] Unlike other consumption activities, leisure and social activities are also time-intensive. Namely, time investment often accounts for a great proportion of the time and material investment in leisure and social activities. Therefore, leisure and social activities are particularly influenced by people's discretionary time. The length of relatively non-discretionary time for work, housework, child care, etc., can significantly affect the amount of time people spend on leisure and social activities. Compared with children and adolescents, and the elderly, working people with children have relatively less leisure social time; women may have less leisure social time than men because women are the ones who mainly perform household chores and childcare activities.

---

[1] Yan Jiang, "A Study On Urban Residents' Willingness to Invest Leisure Time and Its Influencing Factors—Hangzhou as an Example", *Ecological Economy*, 2012 (3).

F. Du et al., *Chinese People's Time Use and Their Quality of Life*,
https://doi.org/10.1007/978-981-99-5526-8_10

People's education level, income level, and the economic development and infrastructure of the region also affect residents' leisure time and quality.[2] Some scholars have classified leisure activities into four categories: active–passive (watching games, etc.), passive-passive (watching movies, staying at home, etc.), active-active (doing sports, studying, etc.), and passive-active (playing games, etc.). Based on survey data in Shenzhen, it is found that Chinese men prefer active-active leisure, while women prefer passive-passive leisure.[3] Some scholars also classify residents' leisure activities into learning (e.g., reading), fitness (e.g., physical exercise), recreation (e.g., watching TV), and hobbies and social activities (e.g., playing chess, eating).[4]

The level of education affects people's leisure patterns, and the level of income restricts people's choices; due to the difference in cultural and economic development between urban and rural areas, urban residents have more options for leisure activities than rural residents. Some scholars found that the education level is proportional to the number of people who "exercise regularly", and the main obstacle to residents' participation in physical exercise is also the "lack of time"; in addition, the imbalance of urban and rural economic development also causes the imbalance of involvement in physical fitness activities in urban and rural areas.[5] Some scholars also found regional differences in residents' reading activities: urban residents read more than rural residents, and people in economically developed regions read more than people in other regions.[6]

This chapter uses data from the 2017 Chinese Time Use Survey to analyze social differences in leisure and social activities among Chinese residents in terms of gender, urban and rural differences, city-to-city differences, age, education level, and household income level. Socioeconomic development will bring about changes and upgrades in residents' leisure and social activities. Accordingly, the consumption market of leisure will also change. Understanding the situation of leisure and social activities of Chinese residents and studying the differences between different groups of people have far-reaching implications for formulating appropriate industrial policies, promoting the industrial development of leisure and social activities, improving the life quality of residents, and promoting the sustainable and healthy development of the national economy.

The interviewees of the 2017 Chinese Time Use Survey were residents aged three years and above, with a total sample size of 30,604 people. Removing the samples with incomplete basic information, the sample size available for analysis in this

[2] Yong Zhou, "Time Allocation Factors in The Development of National Leisure Industry", *Finance & Economics*, 2012 (5).

[3] Lingfei Wu, "Research on Urban Residents' Leisure Satisfaction Based on Leisure Type", *Statistics & Decision*, 2013 (24).

[4] An'min Zhang, "Research on the Influence Mechanism of Residents' Leisure Participation in China", *Human Geography*, 2013 (28).

[5] Chongmin Jiang, Yanfeng Zhang, Rui Cai, Yimin Zhang, Mei Wang, Yazheng Meng, Ming Zhang, Jinhui Zou, "Analysis of the Current Situation of Chinese Urban and Rural Residents' Participation in Physical Exercise in 2007", *China Sports Science*, 2009 (3).

[6] Juying Qiao, Ruiping Li, "Analysis of the Current National Reading Situation in China", *Library and Information Service*, 2009 (13).

chapter is 29,254 people, including 19,157 in urban areas and 10,097 in rural areas; 14,971 men and 14,283 women.

Classification of Leisure and Social Activities

According to the activity classification of the 2017 Chinese Time Use Survey, leisure and social activities include three major categories: physical exercise and fitness activities, recreation and leisure, and social interaction and religious activities. For convenience, this chapter refers to physical exercise and fitness activities as physical fitness, social interaction and religious activities as social activities. This chapter further divides the three categories of activities, as shown in Table 10.1.

As shown in Table 10.1, this chapter defines physical fitness, reading, and hobbies as active leisure or high-quality leisure; watching TV and resting are defined as passive leisure or low-quality leisure. Physical fitness, reading, and hobbies require active participation. These activities are good for physical and mental health, and life enrichment. They can be regarded as some human capital investment. Therefore, this chapter regards them as active leisure/high-quality leisure. In contrast, watching TV and resting often do not require active participation; therefore, this chapter regards them as passive/low-quality leisure.

Social interactions positively affect the formation of individuals' social capital and the harmonious development of society. Social interactions include face-to-face socializing, non-face-to-face socializing, and religious activities, among which the average participation length of face-to-face socializing is higher than that of non-face-to-face socializing and religious activities; therefore, this chapter focuses on face-to-face socializing in the analysis of social interactions.

Table 10.1 Classification of leisure and social activities

Physical fitness		
Recreation and leisure	Reading	Active leisure/high-quality leisure
	Hobbies	
	Watching TV	Passive leisure/low-quality leisure
	Resting	
Social interactions	Face-to-face socializing	
	Non-face-to-face socializing	
	Religious activities	

Table 10.2 Average length of leisure and social activities of Chinese residents Unit: hours/day

Activity	National total	Urban	Rural	Male	Female
Active leisure	1.73	1.95	1.41	1.91	1.54
Among which: physical fitness	0.57	0.69	0.39	0.60	0.53
Reading	0.27	0.34	0.17	0.30	0.24
Hobbies	0.89	0.92	0.85	1.01	0.77
Passive leisure	2.32	2.21	2.46	2.36	2.28
Among which: watching TV	1.70	1.68	1.73	1.75	1.65
Resting	0.62	0.53	0.73	0.61	0.63
Social interactions	0.50	0.45	0.57	0.48	0.52
Among which: face-to-face socializing	0.44	0.38	0.52	0.42	0.45

General Information

Overview

Table 10.2 reports the time use status of leisure and social activities of Chinese residents in 2017.

The average length of active leisure (including physical fitness, reading, and hobbies) was 1.73 h per day, higher in urban areas than in rural areas at 1.95 h and higher for men than women. The average length of passive leisure (including watching TV and resting) was 2.32 h per day, slightly higher in rural than urban areas and somewhat higher for men than women. The average length of social interaction was 0.50 h per day, of which face-to-face socializing accounted for 88%. The average length of face-to-face socializing was higher in rural areas than in urban areas and slightly higher for women than men.

Comparison with 2008

China's economy has grown considerably in the past decade, and residents' income and living standards have also increased substantially. To understand the changes in leisure and social activities of Chinese residents over time, this chapter compares the 2017 results with the data in the *2008 Compilation of Time Use Survey Information* published by the Department of Social and Science and Technology Statistics, National Bureau of Statistics.[7] This is shown in Fig. 10.1.

[7] *The 2008 Compilation of Time Use Surveys* samples are from Chinese residents aged 15–74 in 10 provinces (cities). For comparability, this subsection selects samples of the same age group from the same 10 provinces (cities) in the 2017 Chinese Time Use Survey for calculation. In addition, "resting" was not included in the 2008 Chinese Time Use Survey, while the option "resting" was added in the 2017 Chinese Time Use Survey.

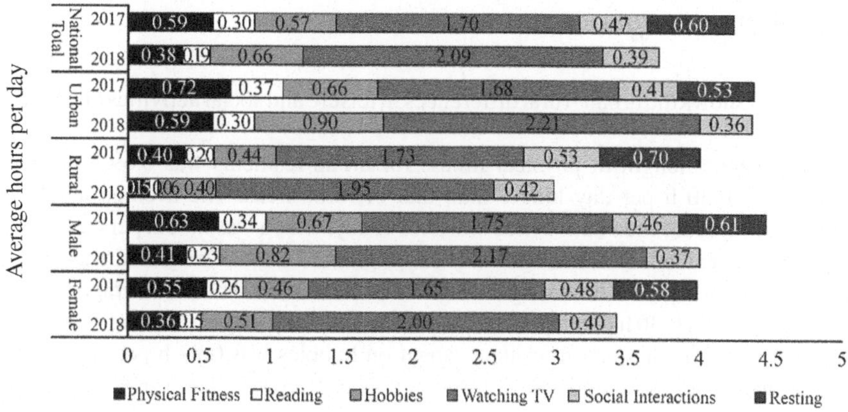

Fig. 10.1 Comparison of the average hours of leisure and social activities of Chinese residents in 2008 and 2017

Figure 10.1 shows that compared with 2008, the average length of leisure and social interaction of Chinese residents in 2017 increased by 0.52 h per day. The quality of leisure and social interaction also improved: the average length of active leisure activities such as sports and fitness, reading and hobbies increased by 0.23 h per day, and the average length of watching TV as passive leisure decreased by 0.39 h per day.

The urban–rural and gender differences in leisure and social activities have also narrowed compared to 2008. In 2008, the urban–rural difference in the average length of leisure and social activities was 1.38 h per day and the gender difference was 0.58 h per day; in 2017, the urban–rural gap in the average length of leisure and social activities decreased to 0.37 h per day and the gender difference decreased to 0.48 h per day.

In addition, the gap between China and the United States is also narrowing: the average length of leisure and social activities of US residents was 5.09 h per day in 2008, and 4.72 h per day in 2016, a decrease of 0.37 h per day; the average length of leisure and social activities of Chinese residents was 4.20 h per day in 2008, and 4.69 h per day in 2017, an increase of 0.49 h per day.

Urban–Rural Differences and City-to-City Differences

Due to the imbalance of economic development and infrastructure construction between urban and rural areas and different cities in China, there are obvious urban–rural differences and city-to-city differences in leisure and social activities.

Urban–Rural Differences

Table 10.3 shows the urban–rural differences in leisure and social activities of Chinese residents.

The average length of physical fitness for urban residents was 0.69 h per day, which was 0.30 h per day longer than that of rural areas. The average length of physical fitness for men nationwide was 0.60 h/day, which was 0.07 h per day longer than that of women. The average daily reading time of urban residents was 0.34 h per day, which was one time longer than that of rural areas, and the average reading time of men was 0.30 h per day, which was 0.06 h per day longer than that of women. The average time that urban residents spent on hobbies was 0.92 h per day, 0.07 h longer than rural areas, and 1.01 h for men, which were 0.24 h per day longer than women.

Urban residents spent an average of 1.68 h per day watching TV, which was 0.05 h shorter than that in rural areas. The national average length of TV watching for men was 1.75 h per day, 0.10 h longer than that for women. The average time spent by urban residents for rest was 0.53 h per day, 0.20 h shorter than that of rural areas. The national average length of rest for men was 0.61 h per day, 0.02 h shorter than for women.

The average daily length of social interactions of urban residents was 0.45 h per day, which was 0.12 h per day shorter than that of rural areas, and of which the average daily length of face-to-face socializing (chatting) of urban residents was 0.38 h per day, which was 0.14 h per day shorter than that of rural areas. The average length of social activities for men nationwide was 0.48 h per day, which was 0.04 h per day shorter than for women. The average length of face-to-face socializing for men nationwide was 0.42 h per day, which was 0.03 h per day shorter than for women.

Figure 10.2 shows the types of leisure activities in urban and rural areas.

It can be seen that the leisure activities of urban and rural residents were still dominated by passive leisure. The average participation length was higher for men

Table 10.3 Urban–rural differences in leisure and social interaction of Chinese residents Unit: hours/day

Activity	China			Urban			Rural		
	Total	Male	Female	Total	Male	Female	Total	Male	Female
Physical fitness	0.57	0.60	0.53	0.69	0.72	0.65	0.39	0.43	0.36
Reading	0.27	0.30	0.24	0.34	0.38	0.30	0.17	0.20	0.15
Hobbies	0.89	1.01	0.77	0.92	1.05	0.77	0.85	0.94	0.76
Watching TV	1.70	1.75	1.65	1.68	1.71	1.63	1.73	1.79	7.68
Resting	0.62	0.61	0.63	0.53	0.52	0.55	0.73	0.73	0.73
Social interactions	0.50	0.48	0.52	0.45	0.43	0.47	0.57	0.56	0.59
Among which: face-to-face socializing	0.44	0.42	0.45	0.38	0.37	0.40	0.52	0.51	0.53

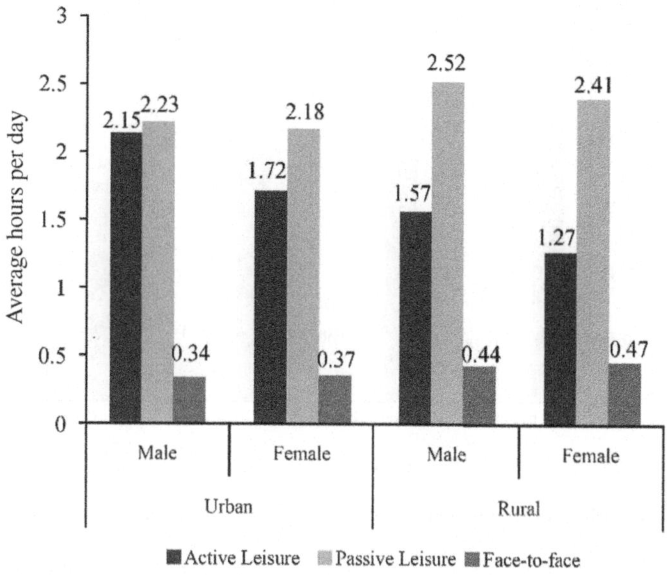

Fig. 10.2 Comparison of the quality of leisure and social activities between urban and rural residents in China

than women in urban and rural areas. Combining the information in Table 10.3, it can be seen that watching TV took up the most time among the passive leisure activities. The longest average time spent watching TV per day was 1.79 h per day by rural male residents. As data shows, it is not women who are more interested in watching TV. Among active leisure activities, time spent on physical fitness and reading was longer in urban than rural areas. This situation may be due to several reasons: first, the lack of supporting facilities for leisure and social activities in rural areas compared to urban ones; second, the lower education level of rural residents compared to urban ones, which limited activities like reading; third, the more physical labor in rural areas compared to towns, which made rural residents more willing to watch TV, rest and do other such activities instead of physical fitness, especially for rural women.

According to the 2017 Chinese Time Use Survey data, although cell phones and social platforms binding phone numbers (such as WeChat) have become essential tools for residents to communicate daily, direct face-to-face socializing was still the most important way of social interaction. The average length of direct face-to-face socializing was higher in rural areas than in urban ones. The average length of face-to-face socializing per day was higher for women than for men. Although direct face-to-face socializing was still the most important way of social interaction, among non-face-to-face socializing, the participation rate of social activities via WeChat occupied the first place and became the primary method. The participation rate was higher in urban than rural areas, and higher of women than that men.

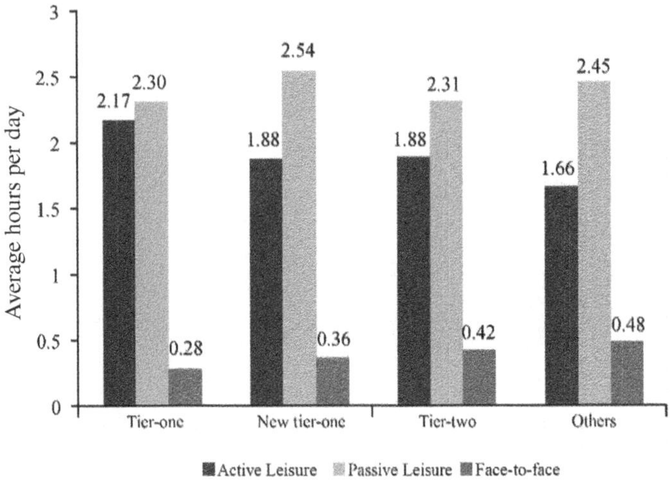

Fig. 10.3 Comparison of leisure and social activities of residents in different types of cities in China

City-to-City Differences

According to the different development degrees, Chinese cities can be divided into tier-one, new tier-one, tier-two, etc.[8] The differences in leisure and social activities in various types of towns are shown in Fig. 10.3.

It can be seen that the more developed the city is, the longer the active leisure time and the shorter the face-to-face socializing time of residents are. The relationship between passive leisure and city type is not obvious.

[8] City classification is shown in the *2017 China City Business Attractiveness Ranking: What Makes the Best Cities* published by China Business Network on May 25, 2017. This ranking divides 338 cities in the Chinese mainland into 4 tier-one cities, 15 new tier-one cities, 30 tier-two cities, and several tier-three, four, and five cities. The four tier-one cities are Beijing, Shanghai, Guangzhou and Shenzhen. The 15 new tier-one cities are Chengdu, Hangzhou, Wuhan, Chongqing, Nanjing, Tianjin, Suzhou, Xi'an, Changsha, Shenyang, Qingdao, Zhengzhou, Dalian, Dongguan, and Ningbo. And the 30 tier-two cities are Xiamen, Fuzhou, Wuxi, Hefei, Kunming, Harbin, Jinan, Foshan, Changchun, Wenzhou, Shijiazhuang, Nanning, Changzhou, Quanzhou, Nanchang Guiyang, Taiyuan, Yantai, Jiaxing, Nantong, Jinhua, Zhuhai, Huizhou, Xuzhou, Haikou, Urumqi, Shaoxing, Zhongshan, Taizhou, and Lanzhou.

Differences in Leisure and Social Activities of Residents of Different Ages

Residents of different ages are at different stages of their lives, and thus their leisure and social activities vary. Table 10.4 and Fig. 10.4 show the leisure and social activities of Chinese residents in different age groups.

In active leisure, the average hours of physical fitness were longer for the older groups from the age of 50 onward. What is more obvious is that after the age of 50, the increase in physical fitness hours was greater for men compared to women, leading to a widening gender difference. The duration of physical fitness was shorter for high school students and longer for college students. The average time residents spent on reading activities each day was less. The longest average reading hours were concentrated in the age group of 18–21 years old, which was 0.66 h per day. The average hours spent on reading activities per day were longer for women than men below the age of 30, and longer for men than women above the age of 30. The gender difference widened. Regarding hobbies, the longer average hours were concentrated in the 18–21 age group, and the average hours spent on hobbies dropped significantly after the age of 30 when people started a family.

The average hours spent watching TV increased as people became older. In the three groups of 15–30 years old, women watched TV longer than men, and after 30 years old, men watched TV longer than women. The duration of rest increased with growing age, with little gender difference.

Regarding differences in leisure and social activities, the overall trend was that young people spent less time on leisure and social activities and older people spent more. In Fig. 10.4, residents' average daily time spent on leisure and social activities tended to increase significantly after age 50. It was generally higher for men than for women. From the figure, it can be observed that after age 60, the gender difference widened, although the average length of leisure social activities increased for both men and women. As seen in other chapters, the increase in women's activities in caring for the third generation and other family members during this period may increase women's unpaid labor in this age group, thus making the gender gap widen. This situation was more pronounced in rural areas.

It is also evident from Fig. 10.4 that the length of leisure and social activities was significantly longer for residents aged 18–21 than for those aged 12–17, reflecting the difference in leisure and social activities between the university level and the high school level.

There was a significant lack of physical fitness among primary and secondary school students, as shown in Fig. 10.5.

The Ministry of Education's *Regulations on the Work Concerning Physical Education and Sport in Schools* stipulates that students are guaranteed one hour of physical activity per day. Based on data from the 2017 Chinese Time Use Survey, Fig. 10.5 shows that elementary and senior high school students had less than one hour of physical exercise and fitness activity. In the age group of high school students (15–17 years old), the average hours of physical exercise and fitness activities on weekdays were

Table 10.4 Average length of leisure and social activities of Chinese residents of different ages Unit: hours/day

Age groups	Physical fitness		Reading		Hobbies		Watching TV		Resting		Social interactions	
	Male	Female	Male	Female	Male	Female	Male	Female	Male	Female	Male	Female
3–5	0.22	0.25	0.05	0.09	4.65	4.61	1.84	1.77	0.24	0.30	0.13	0.23
6–8	0.21	0.21	0.06	0.10	1.94	2.28	2.02	1.38	0.26	0.30	0.09	0.20
9–11	0.16	0.19	0.11	0.14	1.34	1.25	1.46	1.42	0.26	0.25	0.24	0.16
12–14	0.36	0.23	0.27	0.29	1.16	0.64	1.41	1.28	0.27	0.39	0.24	0.16
15–17	0.31	0.18	0.44	0.41	1.32	0.58	0.86	1.08	0.34	0.32	0.36	0.40
18–21	0.46	0.40	0.63	0.70	1.93	0.94	0.83	1.08	0.42	0.44	0.59	0.48
22–30	0.47	0.34	0.49	0.50	1.29	0.63	0.94	1.25	0.43	0.33	0.48	0.32
31–40	0.33	0.37	0.37	0.29	0.52	0.37	1.31	1.29	0.49	0.40	0.37	0.33
41–50	0.33	0.37	0.31	0.17	0.30	0.35	1.65	1.62	0.63	0.57	0.41	0.45
51–60	0.76	0.73	0.20	0.12	0.34	0.38	2.25	2.00	0.61	0.60	0.44	0.51
61–70	1.40	1.09	0.29	0.29	0.42	0.45	2.92	2.30	0.96	1.10	0.56	0.79
71–80	1.58	1.25	0.26	0.14	0.56	0.44	2.94	2.62	1.67	1.54	0.85	0.99
81 and above	1.62	0.80	0.38	0.20	0.51	0.38	2.73	1.97	2.40	2.99	0.85	0.99

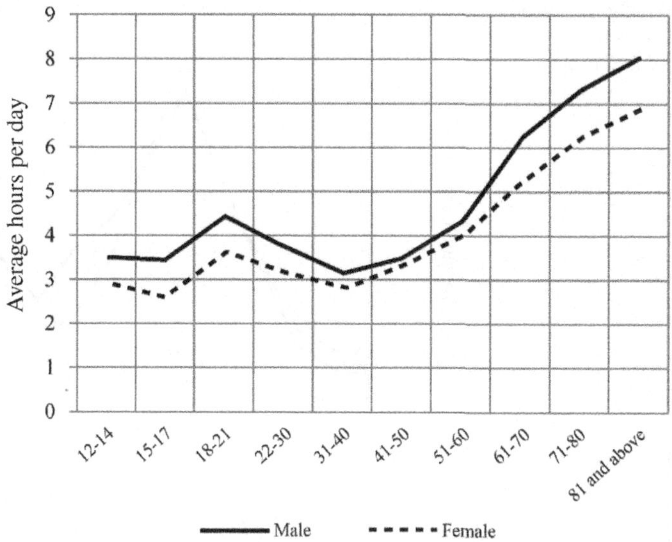

Fig. 10.4 Gender differences in the length of leisure and social activities among residents of different ages

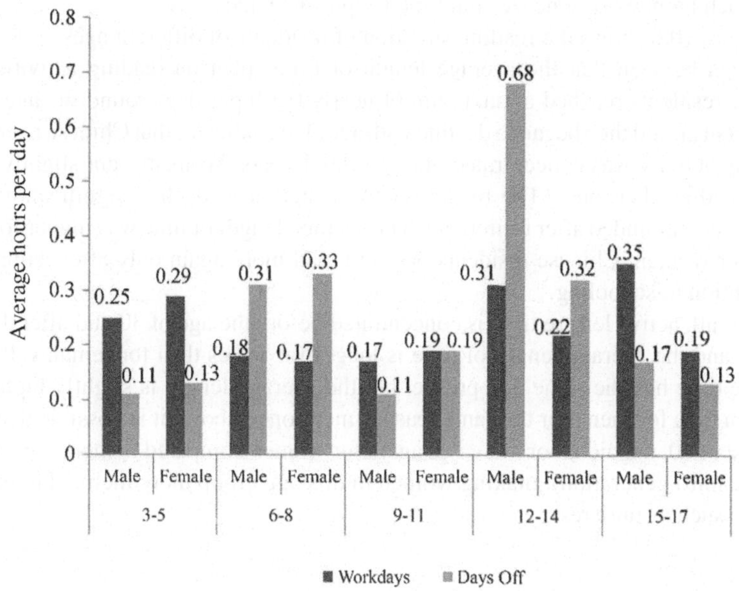

Fig. 10.5 Average hours of physical fitness for primary and secondary school students

Fig. 10.6 Average length of reading activities for residents of different ages

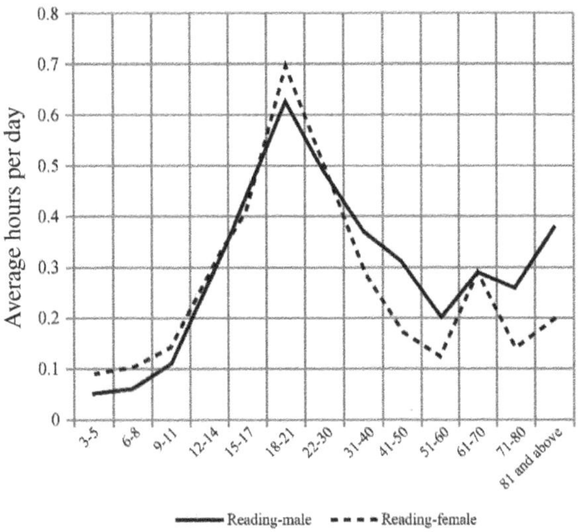

significantly more than the average hours on days off. These can be explained by the fact that senior high school students attend various tutorials on their days off or that too much homework squeezes out time for physical activities.

Figure 10.6 shows the reading situation of residents of different ages.

It can be seen that the average length of time spent on reading activities per day by residents reached a maximum of nearly 0.7 h per day around the age of 20 (university), and then began to decline with age. This indicates that Chinese residents' reading activity was concentrated during school years. Women spent slightly more time reading than men. The reading activity started to decline significantly after work, but rebounded after retirement. The average length of time was higher for men than for women. Chinese residents begin to read more again only after retirement, in addition to schooling.

Overall, active leisure time is concentrated before the age of 30 and after the age of 70, and the average length of time is longer for males than for females. Passive leisure time has the same age profile, but the average length is slightly higher for women than for men. For the same reasons mentioned above, it is possible that after the age of 60, unpaid labor increases again for women compared to men (e.g., caring for the third generation), making women in this age group more inclined to passive leisure such as pure rest.

Differences in Leisure and Social Activities Among Residents with Different Education Levels

Residents with different education levels have different perceptions of the value of leisure and social activities, so the education level affects how people enjoy leisure and social activities. This section analyzes the differences in leisure and social activities of residents with different education levels. In the 2017 Chinese Time Use Survey data, only the sample aged 16 and above provided information on education level, so this section analyzes the residents aged 16 and above.

Table 10.5 shows the overall situation of leisure and social activities among residents with different education levels.

As can be seen, those with lower education levels spent more time on rest and socializing on average. Except for socializing, men spent more time on physical fitness and rest than women. The higher the education level, the longer the average length of reading, but contrariwise, the shorter the time spent watching TV. The gender difference was not significant.

Figure 10.7 shows that the average length of time residents spend reading and watching TV is directly related to their education levels.

The higher the level of education, the longer the time spent on reading per day. Residents who had never gone to school spent an average of 0.03 h/day on reading, while those with bachelor's degrees or above spent nearly 0.70 h/day reading. The average daily reading time of women with college education or above was longer than that of men, and the average daily reading time of men with a college education or below was longer than that of women. In contrast to reading activities, time spent watching TV became less and less as the education level increased. From Fig. 10.7, it can be seen that people with high education levels read for a long time. Reading may also form part of the work for people with high education levels. It may also be due to the fact that recreation and leisure tended to be more active and high-quality for people with higher education compared to those with low education. Also, it can be seen from the two activities, reading and watching TV, that the gender difference was narrowing as the education level climbed.

According to the 2017 Chinese Time Use Survey data, the average length of residents' daily social interaction activities was 0.50 h/day. Among them, the average length of face-to-face socializing was 0.44 h/day. Figure 10.8 shows that a higher education level comes with longer face-to-face socializing and shorter non-face-to-face socializing. Gender differences are not significant.

Overall, the higher the education level, the higher the average length of active leisure and the lower the average length of passive leisure. The gender difference narrowed, but the total leisure time did not increase significantly with the increase in education level.

Table 10.5 Average length of leisure and social activities among Chinese residents with different education levels Unit: hours/day

	Physical fitness		Reading		Hobbies		Watching TV		Resting		Social interactions	
	Male	Female	Male	Female	Male	Female	Male	Female	Male	Female	Male	Female
Unschooled	0.55	0.59	0.04	0.02	1.63	0.74	1.87	1.72	1.31	1.48	0.59	0.84
Elementary school	0.74	0.61	0.11	0.11	0.38	0.31	2.16	1.95	0.99	0.84	0.58	0.59
Junior high school	0.65	0.59	0.30	0.20	0.60	0.50	1.91	1.80	0.62	0.46	0.46	0.43
Senior high school	0.64	0.59	0.39	0.38	0.64	0.52	1.76	1.56	0.49	0.38	0.36	0.40
Technical secondary school/secondary vocational school	0.66	0.67	0.53	0.35	1.01	0.76	1.60	1.72	0.56	0.36	0.56	0.30
Junior college/high vocational school	0.70	0.46	0.53	0.55	1.00	0.55	1.41	1.34	0.46	0.56	0.33	0.35
Undergraduate level	0.73	0.52	0.68	0.64	1.08	0.62	0.98	1.05	0.39	0.42	0.45	0.43
Graduate level	0.47	0.44	0.43	0.88	0.57	0.41	1.00	0.72	0.19	0.12	0.35	0.39

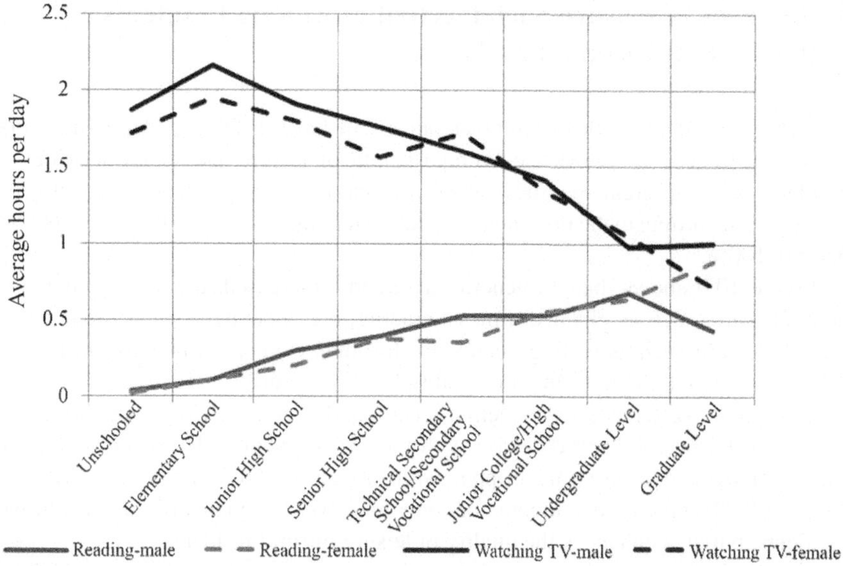

Fig. 10.7 Average length of time spent reading and watching TV by residents with different education levels

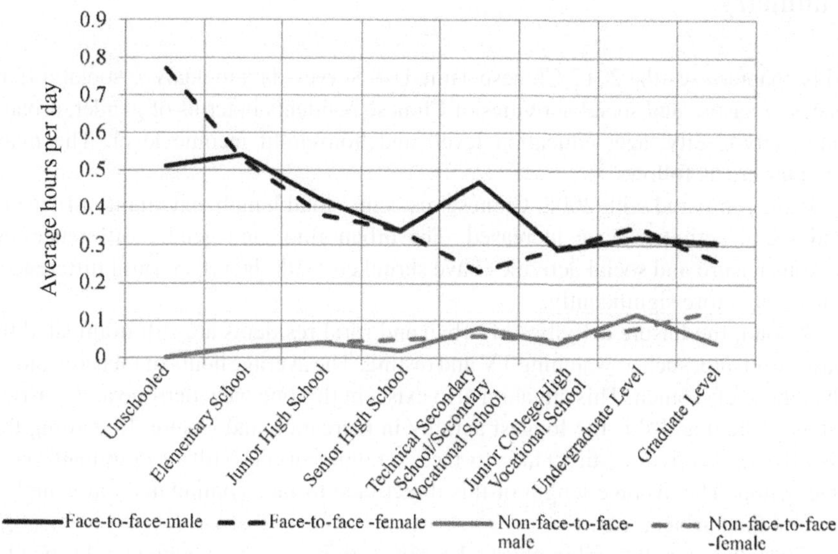

Fig. 10.8 Average length of social interactions of residents with different education levels

Differences in Leisure Social Activities Among Residents with Different Income Levels

Obviously, residents with different incomes will have different leisure and social activities. Table 10.6 shows the average length of leisure and social activities of residents with different incomes, where the income levels are grouped into five categories according to the provincial per capita income: 0–20, 20–40, 40–60, 60–80, and 80–100%.

Figure 10.9 shows that, in general, as income increased, the average hours of active leisure, such as physical fitness, reading, etc. increased, while the hours of passive leisure such as resting decreased. In other words, the increase in income level is conducive to improving the quality level of leisure.

The gender difference in residents' leisure and social activities, whether active or passive leisure, did not decrease with the rise in income. However, as income increased, passive leisure time dropped while urban–rural differences narrowed (see Fig. 10.10). The increase in income not only improves the quality of leisure of urban residents, but also enhances the quality of leisure of rural residents.

Summary

This chapter uses the 2017 Chinese Time Use Survey data to analyze social differences in leisure and social activities of Chinese residents in terms of gender, urban–rural, city-to-city, age, education level, and household income level. The main findings are as follows.

First, compared with 2008, Chinese residents' total length and quality of leisure and social activities have increased. The urban–rural and gender differences in various leisure and social activities have shrunken, with the urban–rural differences narrowing more significantly.

Second, the leisure activities of urban and rural residents are still dominated by passive leisure, such as watching TV and resting. The average hours of men are longer than those of women. This situation also exists in tier-one, new tier-one and tier-two cities. Watching TV is the longest activity in recreation and leisure. Regarding the type of social activities, direct face-to-face communication is still the dominant social interaction. The average length of this direct face-to-face communication is higher in rural than urban areas.

Third, the overall trend in physical fitness activities is that young people spend a short amount of time in physical fitness and older people spend a long amount of time. Among them, there is a clear lack of physical exercise for primary and secondary school students. The Ministry of Education's *Regulations on the Work Concerning Physical Education and Sport in Schools* stipulates that students are guaranteed one hour of physical activity per day. Both elementary and high school students have less than one hour of physical exercise and fitness activities. In the age group of high

Table 10.6 Average length of leisure and social activities of Chinese residents at different income levels Unit: hours/day

Income levels	Physical fitness		Reading		Hobbies		Watching TV		Resting		Social interactions	
	Male	Female	Male	Female	Male	Female	Male	Female	Male	Female	Male	Female
1	0.55	0.59	0.04	0.02	1.63	0.74	1.87	1.72	1.31	1.48	0.59	0.84
2	0.74	0.61	0.11	0.11	0.38	0.31	2.16	1.95	0.99	0.84	0.58	0.59
3	0.65	0.59	0.30	0.20	0.60	0.50	1.91	1.80	0.62	0.46	0.46	0.43
4	0.64	0.59	0.39	0.38	0.64	0.52	1.76	1.56	0.49	0.38	0.36	0.40
5	0.66	0.67	0.53	0.35	1.01	0.76	1.60	1.72	0.56	0.36	0.56	0.30

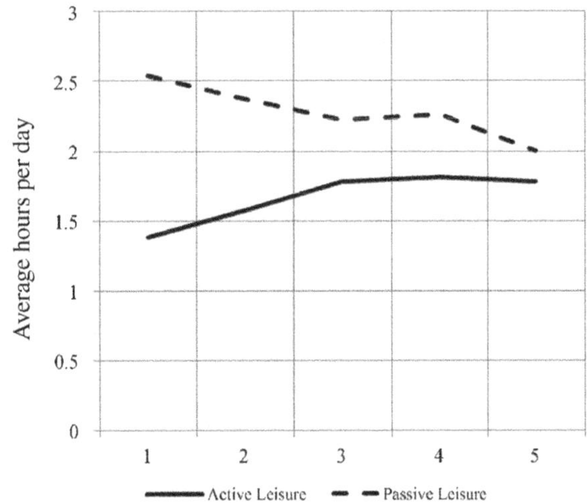

Fig. 10.9 Average length of leisure activities of residents with different income levels

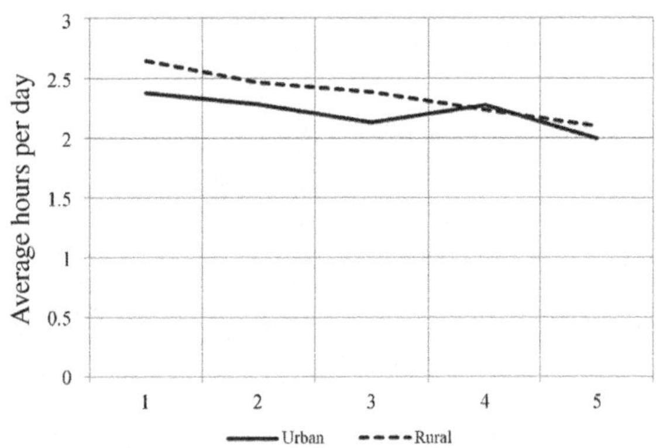

Fig. 10.10 Urban–rural differences in passive leisure of residents with different income levels

school students (15–17 years old), the average hours of physical exercise and fitness activities on weekdays are both significantly more than the average hours on rest days. These can be explained by the fact that high school students attend classes on their days off, or that too much homework squeezes out time for physical activities.

Fourth, the higher the education level, the longer people spend reading and the shorter the time spent watching TV each day. For people with high education levels, reading may also form part of their work. It is also possible that the high education level and the high requirements for human capital investment make the recreation and leisure of this group more inclined to active, high-quality activities. Also, it can be seen from the two activities, reading and watching TV that the gender difference is narrowing as the level of education increases.

The following insights can be drawn from the analysis in this chapter.

Firstly, from the perspective of urban–rural differences in leisure and social activities, considering that the current leisure activities of urban and rural residents are still dominated by passive leisure, such as watching TV, the first thing is to improve the quality of residents' leisure, focusing on the quality of urban and rural TV programs. Second, considering that the time spent on physical labor is higher in rural areas than in urban areas, it is appropriate to increase the facilities and types of leisure and social programs that are more suitable for rural residents' lifestyles. Third, considering the urban residents in tier-one and tier-two economically developed cities, providing them with more leisure time is more important to improve the quality.

Secondly, in terms of age differences in leisure and social activities, the first thing is to provide more leisure and social facilities and programs for the elderly to enrich their leisure and social life, considering that they have more free time. Especially for women, by establishing more and more convenient community family service programs, we can increase their leisure time and improve the life quality in their later years. Second, college students have far more leisure and social time than primary and secondary school students. On one side, it reflects that China's education features "super busy for secondary school students" but "super easy for college students". This phenomenon needs to be adjusted and changed by the country from the policy level.

Thirdly, from the difference in leisure and social activities of residents with different education levels and income levels, education partly determines income. Higher education and income levels lead to more time investment in active leisure, which also means a higher quality of life. Considering that the urban–rural differences in education and income still exist in the short term, the state needs to increase the supply of rural leisure and social activities at the policy level to improve the quality of leisure for rural residents.

Chapter 11
Are the Elderly in China Well-Entertained?

As China gradually enters an aging society, how to make all older people well-raised, well-taken-care-of, well-entertained, and well-secured is drawing more and more attention from society and policymakers.[1] After quitting the labor market, the elderly have more leisure time. Improving the quality of leisure activities can provide a new source of future life and make the elderly's later lives more colorful. For society, the participation of the elderly in leisure with humanistic, cultural, social, and creative aspects can also provide opportunities for individuals to communicate, increase social interaction, develop social homogeneity and promote a harmonious society.[2] Therefore, leisure activities are important for the elderly to live happy lives in their later years.

Using data from the 2017 Chinese Time Use Survey, this chapter analyzes the overall situation of time use of elder people, especially the distribution of leisure time, with the aim of gaining a comprehensive understanding of the distribution of leisure time and leisure content among elder people in China and comparing the allocation of leisure time among different groups of elder people.

Demographic Features and Health Status

The Communiqué of the National Bureau of Statistics of the People's Republic of China on Major Figures of the 2010 Population Census (No. 1) shows that the population aged 65 and above accounts for 8.87% of the total population of China. *The Population Aging and Its Socio-Economic Consequences* published by the United Nations in 1956 writes that if the proportion of elderly people aged 60 and above in

---

[1] Yunpeng Li, "Older People Need Financial Support to Be Well-raised", *People's Tribune*, 2018 (4).

[2] Yongming Wang, "Research on Leisure and Cultural Life of the Elderly in the Context of Aging—Take Changshu as an Example," *Changbai Journal*, 2015 (5).

F. Du et al., *Chinese People's Time Use and Their Quality of Life*,
https://doi.org/10.1007/978-981-99-5526-8_11

Table 11.1 Distribution of sample observations Unit: people

	The young-old		The old		The old-old	
	Urban	Rural	Urban	Rural	Urban	Rural
Male	1297	878	611	343	132	59
Female	1436	798	668	318	156	83
Total	2733	1676	1279	661	288	142

the total population of a country or region reaches 10%, or the proportion of elderly people aged 65 and above in the total population reaches 7%, it is an aging country or region. China has already entered an aging society based on this standard. Since 2000, the National Bureau of Statistics has been using "65 years old" as the starting age for defining the elderly population.[3] Accordingly, this chapter defines the population aged 65 and above as the elderly. In order to have a clearer understanding of the time allocation of the elderly in different periods, this chapter divides the elderly into three age groups: the young-old (65–74 years old), the old (75–84 years old), and the old-old (85 years old and above), whose sample distribution is shown in Table 11.1.

Demographic Features

The residence status of the elderly in this chapter includes two types: living alone and non-living alone. Living alone means that the elderly do not live with their children or relatives or friends, and non-living alone is the opposite. The marital status of the elderly as married, cohabiting and remarried are referred to as living with a spouse, while unmarried, separated, divorced and widowed are referred to as living without a spouse. Table 11.2 shows that the rate of living alone was higher among the young-old and the old in rural than in urban areas, and the rate of living alone was higher among the old in urban than in rural areas. In terms of the marital status of the elderly, the proportion of rural elderly who did not live with a spouse was higher than that of urban elderly, and the proportion of those who did not live with a spouse increased significantly as they grew older. In addition, the overall education level of the elderly was low, and the education level was mainly concentrated in elementary school and below. The older the age group was, the more concentrated the education level was in the low level. This trend was more obvious in rural areas.

[3] Shenghui Yang, Yong Zhao, Jie Lin, "A Little Reflection on the Criteria for Defining the Elderly Population in China", *Northwest Population Journal*, 2017 (3).

Table 11.2 Demographic features of the elderly Unit: %

		The young-old		The old		The old-old	
		Urban	Rural	Urban	Rural	Urban	Rural
Residence status	Living alone	13.9	17.8	18.6	20.4	13.5	12.0
	Non-living alone	86.1	82.2	81.4	79.6	86.5	88.0
Marital status	Living with a spouse	86.3	84.7	69.2	63.4	42.3	33.1
	Not living with a spouse	13.7	15.3	30.8	36.6	57.7	66.9
Education level	Unschooled	13.0	33.4	21.5	48.5	45.8	70.0
	Elementary school	32.4	47.6	30.5	38.9	21.5	26.4
	Junior high school	30.9	15.1	17.3	9.4	13.7	3.6
	Senior high school	15.8	3.6	17.2	3.0	9.2	0.0
	College and above	7.9	0.3	13.6	0.2	9.9	0.0

Health Status

Health affects the way the elderly live and use their time. Table 11.3 shows that the rate of no disease decreased with age, while the opposite was true for the rate of those physically challenged. The rate of the elderly with two or more diseases was about 30% in all three age groups. The overall participation rate in social health insurance was higher among the elderly.

Time Allocation of the Elderly

Based on the data from the 2017 Chinese Time Use Survey, this chapter divides the overall time use of the elderly into four major categories: paid labor, unpaid labor, leisure and social activities, and self-care. Paid labor mainly includes work and household production and operation; unpaid labor mainly includes housework, caring for adults and minors, etc.; leisure and social activities include reading, playing games, watching TV, doing sports and fitness, joining in various types of face-to-face

Table 11.3 Health status of the elderly Unit: %

Group	The young-old		The old		The old-old	
	Urban	Rural	Urban	Rural	Urban	Rural
No disease	16.2	22.7	15.3	17.9	12.9	13.4
The rate of those physically challenged	1.9	4.2	3.7	7.0	4.2	5.6
Suffering from two or more diseases	26.7	30.3	29.6	28.3	26.4	30.3
Protected by social health insurance	95.1	94.4	92.0	91.8	90.4	87.9

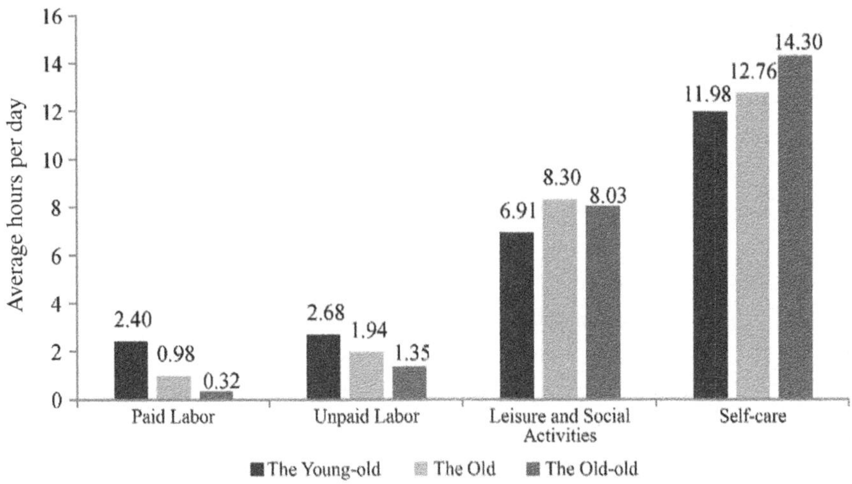

Fig. 11.1 Comparison of the four types of time allocation for the elderly

interactions and non-face-to-face interactions; self-care includes activities such as sleeping, personal hygiene, and eating.

Figure 11.1 shows the time allocation of the elderly in a day. As can be seen, the average participation length of activities in a day for the elderly were, in descending order, self-care, leisure and social activities, unpaid labor, and paid labor. As the age increased, the time spent on self-care increased but the time spent on paid and unpaid labor decreased. In terms of leisure and social activities, the old spent the most time, followed by the old-old, and the young-old spent the least time. Relatively speaking, the young-old had to take more paid and unpaid labor.

Figure 11.2 shows the urban–rural differences in the activity arrangement of the elderly throughout a day. It can be seen that regardless of age, self-care time and labor time[4] were higher in rural areas than in urban areas. Leisure and social time was higher in urban than in rural areas.

Figure 11.3 shows the gender differences in the arrangement of activities in a day for the elderly. It can be seen that among the elderly, women had more self-care time and unpaid labor time than men, while men had more leisure and social activities and paid labor time than women. The gender difference in self-care time increased with growing age, and the gender difference in leisure and social activities, paid labor and unpaid labor time decreased.

[4] Labor time: refers to the sum of paid and unpaid labor time.

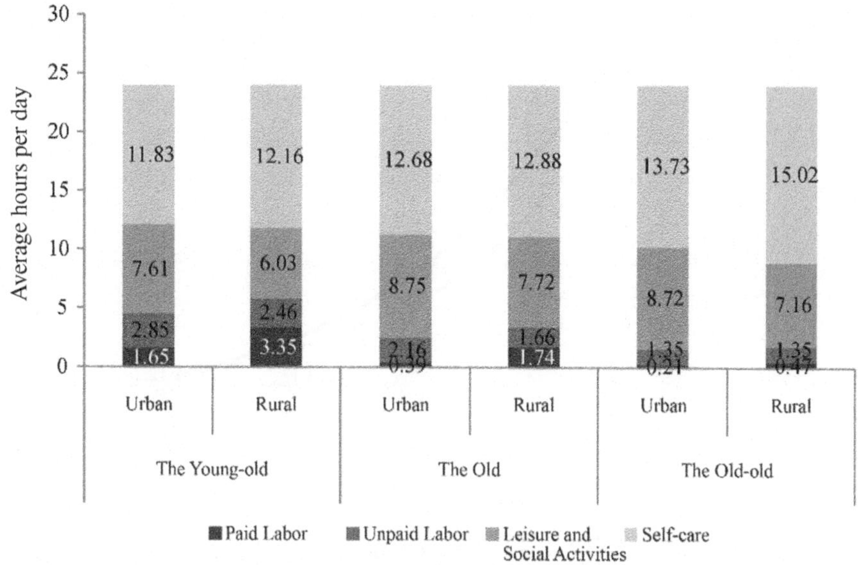

Fig. 11.2 Urban–rural comparison of time allocation of the elderly

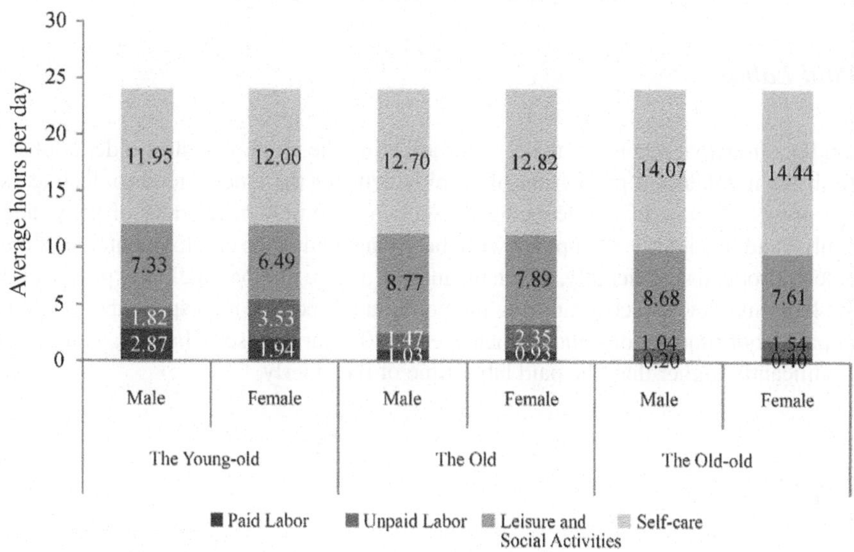

Fig. 11.3 Gender comparison of time allocation of the elderly

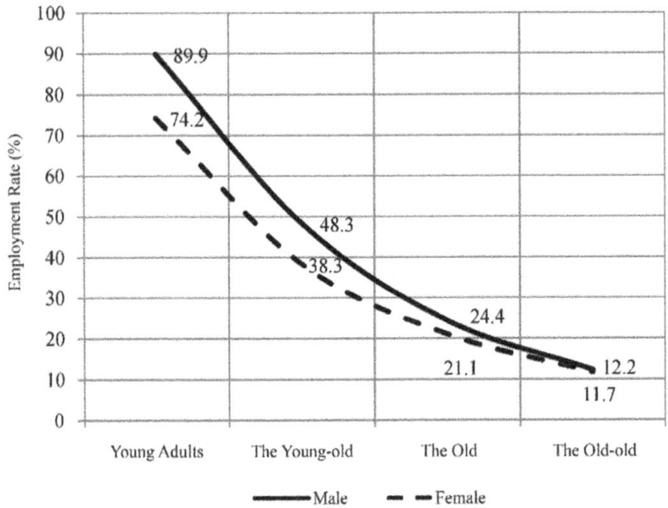

Fig. 11.4 Comparison of employment rates of young adults and the elderly

Distribution of Labor Time Among the Elderly

Paid Labor

Studies show that age is the main factor affecting the employment of older adults.[5] Both the number and proportion of employment for the elderly tend to decline as age grows.[6] Figure 11.4 reflects the changes in the employment rates of the young adults[7] and the elderly. Compared with the young adults, the employment rate of the elderly dropped significantly, which means that a large number of elderly people quit the labor market. Moreover, during the young-adult period, men spent about 7.34 h of paid labor time per day and women spent 5.20 h per day (see Chap. 5), which was significantly higher than the paid labor time of the elderly.

Unpaid Labor

Figure 11.5 shows that, from young adults to the elderly, the duration of unpaid labor for men shows an inverted U-shape, with the young-old at the peak and the

[5] Zugen Zhou, "Analysis of the Employment Situation and Trends of the Elderly Population in Shanghai", *South China Population*, 1993 (2).

[6] Miaohua Lai, "When Will the Party Rest?—Cohort Analysis of Employment Participation of Older People in China", *Social Science of Beijing*, 2017 (3).

[7] Young adults refer to the population aged 22–64 years old.

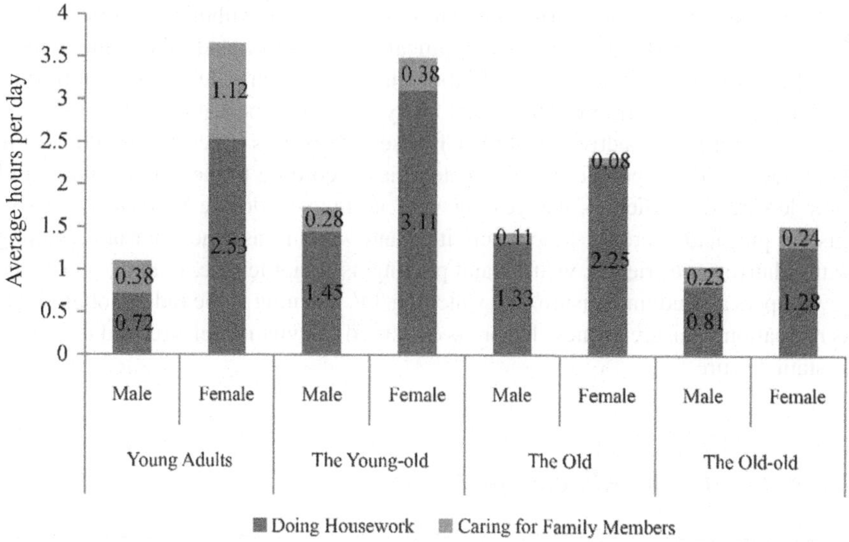

Fig. 11.5 Comparison of unpaid labor between young adults and the elderly

old-old at the bottom; the length of unpaid labor for women shows a straight line downward trend, with female young adults taking up the most unpaid labor and female young-old taking up slightly less unpaid labor than the former. Regardless of the time period, women's unpaid labor time was higher than men's, but the gender difference decreased with growing age.

Leisure Activities of the Elderly

Leisure is important for improving the life quality of the elderly. Leisure activities are not only for killing time, but also for further personal development and improvement, which can enhance interactions with friends and family, provide a new experience, and are especially important to promote physical and mental health.[8] The elderly with higher life satisfaction tend to be those who participate in various leisure activities the most. Leisure activities are beneficial to the physical and psychological development of the elderly.[9]

[8] Tinsley, H. E. A. Teaff, J. D., Clobs, S. L. et al., "N. A System for Classifying Leisure Activities in Terms of the Psychological Benefits of Participation Reported by Older Persons", *Journal of Gerontology*, 1985, (40).

[9] Bevil, Catherine A., O'Connor, Priscilla C., Mattoon, Pamela M., "Leisure Activity, Life Satisfaction, and Perceived Health Status in Older Adults", *Gerontology & Geriatrics Education*, 14(2), 1993.

From the previous comparison, it can be seen that the withdrawal of the elderly from the labor market has led to a significant decrease in paid labor time, which, together with the decline in unpaid labor time, has given older people more time for leisure activities. In order to further analyze the distribution of leisure time and the content of leisure activities of the Chinese elderly, this paper divides the leisure activities of elderly people into five categories according to the actual situation of their leisure life: idleness and resting with nothing to do are defined as passive leisure, physical exercise, fitness activities and walking as fitness leisure, chatting with relatives and friends, visiting and playing as social leisure, reading books and newspapers as studying leisure, and watching TV, listening to the radio, hobbies, etc. as recreational leisure. Fitness leisure is classified as dynamic leisure, and the others as static leisure.

Overview of Time Allocation

Table 11.4 reports the participation rate and average length of leisure activities of the elderly. In terms of leisure status, Chinese elderly people's leisure was mainly static leisure, especially recreational leisure, which occupied the most important position in elderly people's leisure activities. Its participation rate was the highest among all leisure activities. This research conclusion was consistent with Ding Zhihong's[10] research findings. The other static leisure activities, in descending order of participation rate, are passive leisure, social leisure and study leisure. The participation rate of dynamic leisure was higher among the young-old and the old, second only to recreational leisure.

In terms of the length of leisure activities, recreational leisure time was the longest, with all three age groups spending more than 3 h/day on this leisure activity; studying leisure time was the shortest, with the young-old spending only 0.16 h per day. With the increase in age, the leisure time of the fitness and recreational type climbed and then dropped, while the time of passive and social leisure kept increasing, among which, the passive leisure time inclined more and exceeded the fitness among the old and the old-old.

Urban–Rural Differences

There are obvious urban–rural differences in the distribution of leisure time among the elderly, with urban elderly spending more time on leisure than rural elderly, especially on recreational, fitness and studying leisure. On the contrary, the time spent on passive leisure (leisure/rest) was significantly higher in rural than in urban

[10] Zhihong Ding, "Analysis and Reflection on the Characteristics of Leisure Activities of the Elderly in China", *Lanzhou Academic Journal*, 2010 (9).

Table 11.4 Participation rate and the average length of leisure activities of the elderly group

Group	Participation rate (%)					Average hours per day				
	Passive	Social	Recreational	Fitness	Studying	Passive	Social	Recreational	Fitness	Studying
The young-old	35.0	23.1	77.6	45.3	6.6	1.22	0.81	3.41	1.26	0.16
The old	44.0	23.4	73.3	49.6	9.5	2.03	0.91	3.55	1.48	0.25
The old-old	51.5	24.3	58.6	33.1	9.0	2.81	0.95	3.07	0.88	0.25

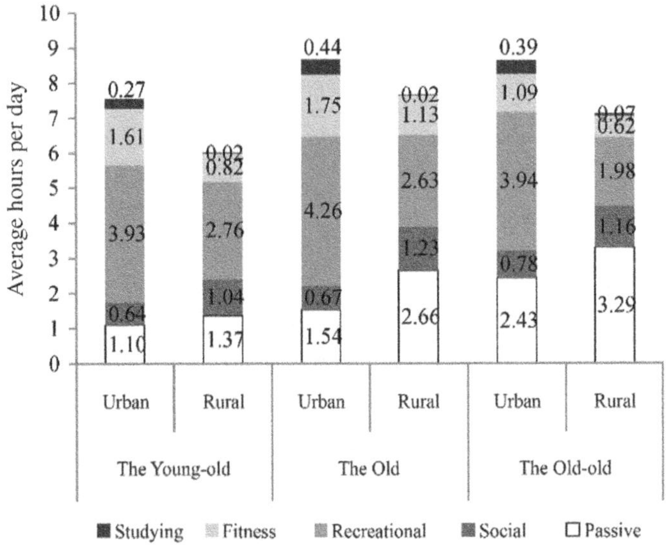

Fig. 11.6 Comparison of leisure activities between the urban and rural elderly

areas; the time spent on social leisure was also the case. This indicates that urban older adults have a higher quality of leisure. For the elderly, the urban–rural differences in various types of leisure time are shown by the fact that as the age increases, the time spent on fitness leisure decreases, the time spent on leisure-oriented leisure increases, and the time spent on studying, social and passive leisure increases first and then decreases (Fig. 11.6).

The time spent on leisure activities by urban and rural elderly people reflects the difference in socioeconomic development between urban and rural areas. The lower level of economic security and fewer facilities for recreational activities in rural areas,[11] and the longer working hours of rural elderly also crowd out leisure time to some extent.

Gender Differences

In terms of gender, as shown in Fig. 11.7, women in the elderly group spent slightly more time on passive and social leisure than men, and less time on pastime, fitness and study leisure than men. In other words, women spent more time than men on lounging and chatting with neighbors and friends, while men spent more time watching TV, walking, doing physical exercise, and reading newspapers. This reflects that female older adults are more willing to participate in group activities than males, while

[11] Lili Wang, "Analysis of the Leisure Activity Participation Status of Chinese Elderly and Its Influencing Factors", *Northwest Population Journal*, 2010 (3).

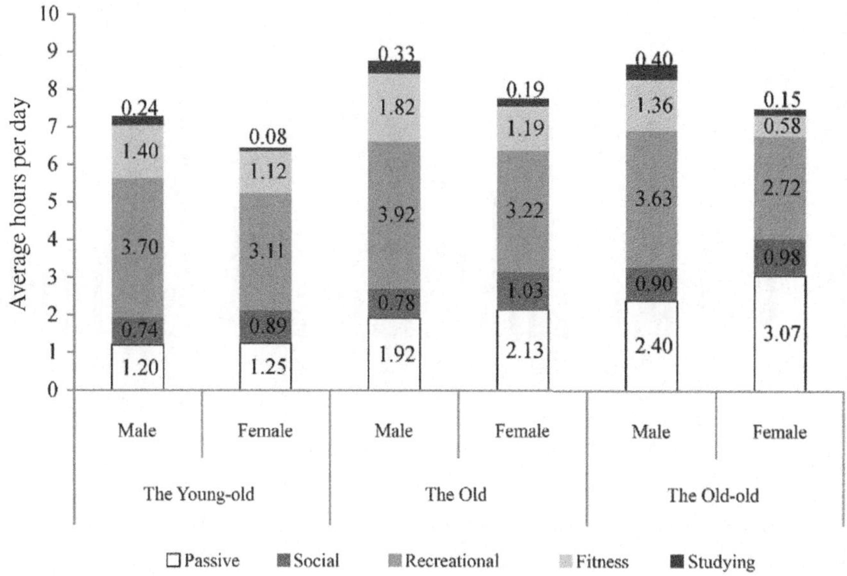

Fig. 11.7 Gender differences in leisure activities of the elderly

male older adults are more willing to participate in activities with more interest and individuality. The gender difference in passive, recreational and fitness leisure time increased with age, the gender difference in social leisure time decreased with age, and the gender gap in study leisure was the largest among the elderly.

Differences in Time Use Among Older Adults with Different Education Levels

Differences in the education levels of the elderly also have an impact on their leisure activities. Figure 11.8 shows that the elderly with low education levels spent more time on passive and social leisure, but less time on recreational, fitness and studying leisure, while the opposite was true for older adults with high education levels. In particular, studying leisure time was directly proportional to the elderly's education level. Those with junior high school level and above spent significantly more time on studying leisure than those with elementary school level or below.

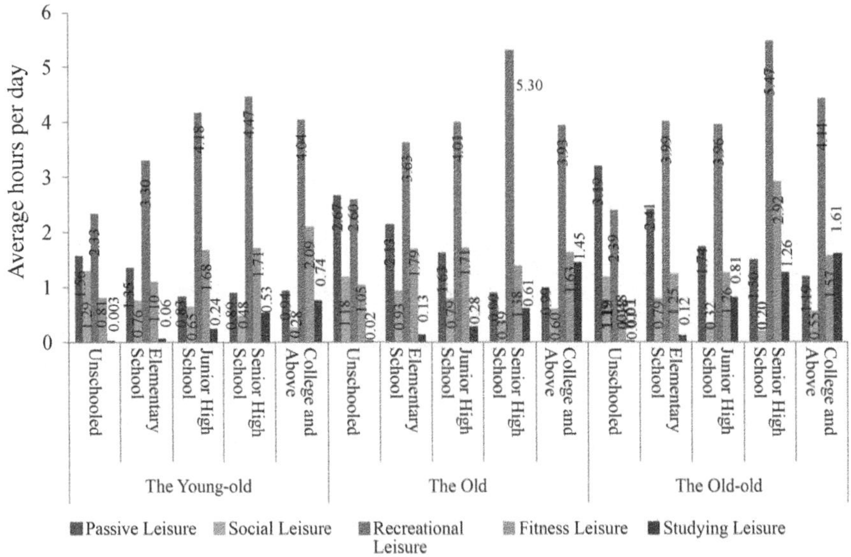

Fig. 11.8 Differences in the education level of leisure activities of the elderly

Differences in Time Use Among Older Adults with Different Income Levels

Figure 11.9 reports the impact of differences in income levels[12] on leisure activities of the elderly. As income inclined, passive leisure time declined and learning leisure time increased. The elderly at middle and high-income levels and above spend more time on recreational and fitness leisure than older adults at other income levels. The social leisure time of the young-old shows a U-shape with the increase in income, while the social leisure time of the old and the old-old shows a decreasing trend.

Differences in Time Use Among the Elderly with Different Residence Status

There are differences in the distribution of leisure time among the elderly depending on their residence status. Figure 11.10 reports the statistical results of the leisure time of the elderly with reference to their residence status. The statistical results in the table show that young-old and the old spent more leisure time living alone, and the old-old spent more leisure time in the non-living alone state. This may be because the old-old were able to receive more family care, which allowed them to have more time for leisure activities. Except for the old-old, the elderly living alone

[12] The income level here refers to the per capita household income level.

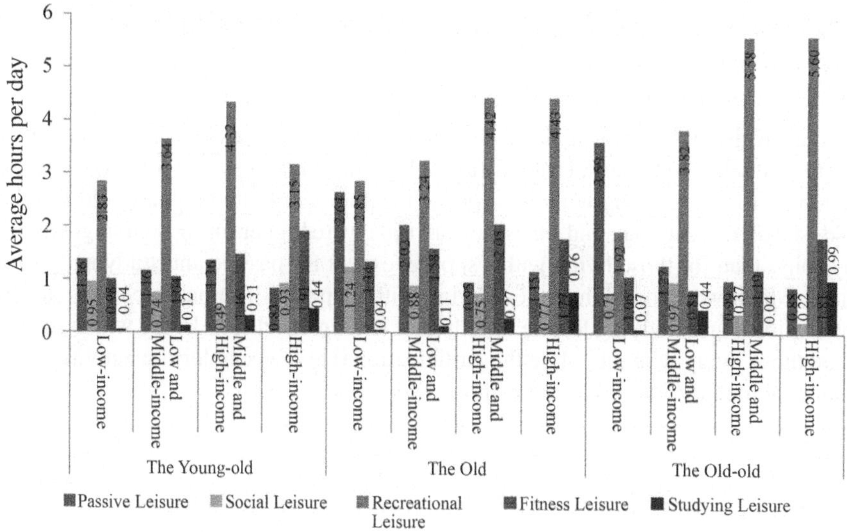

Fig. 11.9 Income level differences in leisure activities for older adults

spent more time on passive leisure, social leisure and studying leisure, while the non-living alone elderly spent more time on recreational leisure. The possible reason for this is that if the elderly are not living alone, they will spend more time caring for others, especially caring for the younger generation. This care-giving time has a crowding-out effect on older adults' social, recreational, and fitness leisure.

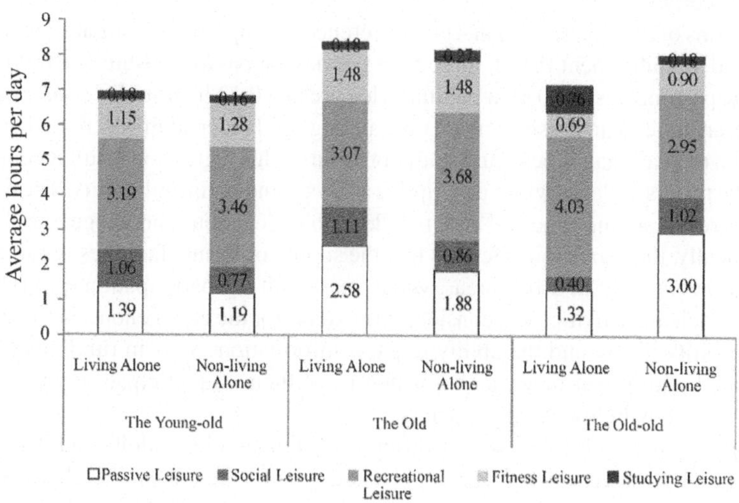

Fig. 11.10 Comparison of residential status of leisure activities among the elderly

Differences in Time Use Among the Elderly with Different Marital Status

There are also differences in the allocation of time for leisure activities among older adults with different marital status. Tables 11.5 and 11.6 show that total leisure time is longer for those living without a spouse together. For both the young-old and the old, social, recreational, and fitness leisure time were higher for those living without a spouse than for those living with a spouse, except for passive and studying leisure time, which were lower than those living with a spouse. The participation rates in recreational and studying leisure were higher among the elderly living with a spouse than those living without, while the participation rate of social leisure activities was higher among the elderly living without a spouse.

Factors Influencing the Leisure Activities of the Elderly

Because urban–rural, gender, income, education level, residential status, and marital status are interrelated and influenced by other factors, to measure the net effect of these group characteristics, an in-depth analysis of the five categories of leisure social activities was conducted using multiple regression, with regression equations controlling for age, gender, region, health, and other factors.

Table 11.7 reports the results of the regression of factors influencing leisure activities of older adults. The table shows that urban/rural, gender, residence status, marital status, education level, and income have significant effects on the leisure activities of the elderly.

In terms of the effect of urban–rural differences, compared with urban older adults, rural older adults spent 0.37 h more time per day on passive leisure and 0.96 h less time on pastime leisure, 0.49 h on fitness leisure and 0.12 h on study leisure. In other words, an increase in passive leisure time among rural older adults decreased the time spent on recreational, fitness, and studying leisure. This regression result is consistent with the results of the previous descriptive analysis, indicating reliability. The reasons for this result are multifaceted and include both endogenous and exogenous factors. Specifically, the exogenous factor is that the supply of leisure facilities in rural areas lags far behind that in urban areas, which may limit the participation of rural older adults in leisure activities to a considerable extent; for the endogenous factor, the gap in the ability to pay and the ability to parse information exists in rural older adults compared with urban older adults, which leads them to participate in passive and social leisure with lower entry barriers.

In terms of the effect of gender differences, female older adults had 0.49 h less leisure time for recreation, 0.23 h less leisure time for fitness, and 0.1 h less leisure time for studying per day compared with male older adults. The reason for this result may be that older women spent more time on family care and household chores. Part of their leisure time was squeezed by unpaid labor.

Table 11.5 Participation rate and average length of leisure activities for living with a spouse

Group	Participation rate (%)					Average hours per day				
	Passive	Social	Recreational	Fitness	Studying	Passive	Social	Recreational	Fitness	Studying
The young-old	35.4	22.3	77.8	45.6	7.0	1.22	0.79	3.41	1.25	0.17
The old	45.7	21.9	75.1	50.1	11.2	2.08	0.86	3.50	1.45	0.31
The old-old	39.9	22.5	64.9	37.5	13.2	1.98	0.55	3.64	1.08	0.43

Table 11.6 Participation rate and average length of leisure activities of living without a spouse

Group	Participation rate (%)					Average hours per day				
	Passive	Social	Recreational	Fitness	Studying	Passive	Social	Recreational	Fitness	Studying
The young-old	33.0	28.2	76.4	43.5	4.1	1.21	0.94	3.44	1.32	0.14
The old	40.1	26.9	69.1	48.3	5.6	1.93	1.03	3.65	1.56	0.13
The old-old	58.7	25.8	55.0	30.6	6.3	3.28	1.23	2.72	0.76	0.13

Table 11.7 Regression results of factors influencing leisure activities of the elderly group

Variables	Passive leisure	Social leisure	Recreational leisure	Fitness leisure	Studying leisure
Sample source (rural = 1, urban = 0)	0.369*** (0.107)	−0.084 (0.077)	−0.961*** (0.136)	−0.490*** (0.088)	−0.121*** (0.047)
Gender (male = 0; female = 1)	−0.152 (0.117)	0.025 (0.084)	−0.491*** (0.149)	−0.234** (0.096)	−0.104** (0.051)
Whether living alone	0.173 (0.125)	0.212** (0.090)	−0.488*** (0.159)	−0.144 (0.103)	0.023 (0.055)
Number of people living in the household	−0.011 (0.023)	0.005 (0.017)	−0.038 (0.030)	−0.039** (0.019)	0.004 (0.010)
Whether living with a spouse	0.011 (0.023)	0.005 (0.017)	−0.038 (0.030)	−0.039** (0.019)	0.004 (0.010)
Education level is elementary school (Yes = 1, No = 0)	−0.365*** (0.134)	−0.101 (0.096)	0.728*** (0.170)	−0.082 (0.110)	0.028 (0.059)
Education level is junior high school (Yes = 1, No = 0)	−0.444*** (0.150)	−0.146 (0.108)	0.7736*** (0.191)	0.199 (0.124)	0.187*** (0.066)
Education level is senior high school (Yes = 1, No = 0)	−0.630*** (0.179)	−0.187 (0.128)	1.042*** (0.226)	0.030 (0.147)	0.539*** (0.078)
Education level is college and above (Yes = 1, No = 0)	−0.609*** (0.209)	−0.191 (0.150)	0.395 (0.265)	0.246 (0.172)	1.042*** (0.091)
Household income is low to middle income group (Yes = 1, No = 0)	−0.133 (0.123)	−0.068 (0.088)	0.347** (0.155)	−0.269*** (0.101)	0.045 (0.053)
Household income is middle to high income group (Yes = 1, No = 0)	−0.365*** (0.127)	−0.177* (0.091)	0.824*** (0.161)	−0.122 (0.105)	0.123** (0.056)
Household income is high income group (Yes = 1, No = 0)	−0.556*** (0.139)	−0.330*** (0.100)	0.911*** (0.176)	0.004 (0.114)	0.246*** (0.061)
Constant term	−2.2258*** (0.682)	0.055 (0.489)	2.236*** (0.864)	2.166*** (0.560)	−0.134 (0.297)
Observed value	3393	3393	3393	3393	3393
R^2	0.076	0.040	0.095	0.082	0.134

Note ① Regression results of control variables are not reported in the table, and the unreported estimation results include health status of the elderly, age, provincial regional dummy variables, and whether they have medical insurance; ② The reference group of education level is the unschooled, and the reference group of household income is low-income level; ③ The numbers in parentheses indicate standard errors; ④ ***, **, **, respectively, indicate that the estimated coefficients pass the significance test at the 1, 5, and 10% levels

The elderly's residence status significantly affects their social and recreational leisure. Compared with non-living alone, those living alone were more likely to spend 0.21 h/day on social leisure activities and 0.48 h/day less on recreational leisure activities; the number of people living with older adults had a significant negative effect on older adults' fitness leisure time; living with a spouse significantly increased older adults' social leisure time.

In terms of education level, the educated elderly spent significantly less time on passive leisure and significantly more time on recreational leisure than the unschooled. The elderly with college or above spent 1.04 h more time on studying leisure per day. In terms of the effect of income, the elderly in high-income households spent 0.55 h less time per day on passive leisure and 0.25 h more time per day on studying leisure. The direction and mechanism of influence of education and income are extremely similar. The elderly with higher education levels (e.g., high school and above) tended to spend less time on passive leisure and more time on studying leisure than those with lower education levels; similarly, older adults in the middle- to high-income or high-income groups tended to spend less time on passive leisure and social leisure and more time on recreational and studying leisure than those in the low-income group. The reason for these results may be that passive leisure and social leisure require lower payment ability and information analysis ability, while studying leisure requires higher payment ability and information collection and analysis ability.

Summary

This chapter uses data from the 2017 Chinese Time Use Survey to interpret the time use of Chinese elderly people and reveal the distribution characteristics, differentiated features, and influencing factors of leisure time of Chinese elderly people. The statistical results show that (1) as older people grow older, paid and unpaid labor time decreases and self-care time increases; (2) Chinese older people's leisure is mainly static, among which recreational leisure occupies the most important position in older people's leisure activities. Its participation rate is the highest among all leisure activities, and its leisure time length is the longest among all leisure activities; (3) in urban areas, older people spend significantly more time on studying, recreational and fitness leisure than in rural areas. In passive and social leisure (leisure/rest), rural areas are significantly higher than urban areas; (4) compared with men, women spend more time on passive and social leisure, and less time on recreation, fitness and learning leisure; (5) as education and income levels increase, older people tend to spend more time on learning leisure, recreation leisure, and fitness leisure, but less time on passive leisure and social leisure; (6) younger older adults who live alone tend to spend more time on passive, social, and learning leisure activities and less time on recreation leisure than those who do not live alone; (7) older adults who live with a spouse are more involved in recreation and learning leisure activities, and those who do not live with a spouse are more involved in social leisure activities.

The results of the above study can bring us the following insights. On the one hand, making the elderly well-entertained is an important part of the balanced development of urban and rural areas, and also an important part of the development of a harmonious society. We should meet the demand for leisure activities of the elderly through infrastructure development and conceptual guidance. On the other hand, policies should not ignore the differences in leisure activity needs between urban and rural areas, income, gender, education level, etc., and prescribe the right medicine for different characteristics of the elderly groups.

Chapter 12
The Chinese Couple

In China, the relationship between a husband and a wife (marriage) is one of the "Five Rites" of Confucianism.[1] *The Book of Rites—Chinese Wedding* explains marriage as follows: "The Chinese Wedding will unite the good of the two families to worship the ancestors, and give life to future generations. Therefore, men of virtue value it". Therefore, traditionally, the relationship between a husband and a wife in China is mainly for the purpose of inheriting the family business and passing on the family blood, and more of a social responsibility. Modern economics considers marriage as an economic and social institution, and the main purpose of marriage and even family existence is to pool resources to obtain a higher level of welfare.[2] However, the specific arrangements of marriage as an economic institution are evolving with economic and social development.[3] The above-mentioned exposition of the relationship between a husband and a wife is more or less too rational and even indifferent. On the other hand, in various literary works of different cultures, we can also see another kind of description of the relationship between a husband and a wife: for example, Su Shi's memorial to his late wife, "ten years, dead and living dim and draw apart. I don't try to remember, but forgetting is hard", the contemporary song, "the most romantic thing I can think of is to grow old with you", the Hollywood movie *Ghost*, which depicts love until death, the Indian epic *Rāmāyaṇa*, and so on. Thus, marriage has a dual attribute: economic function and spiritual companionship. However, it is undeniable that the role of marriage has been changing with the development of productivity and the increase of women's education and labor participation rate.[4]

[1] The other four relationships are that of the monarch and the subjects, the father and the sons, brothers, and friends.

[2] Gary S. Becker, "A Theory of Marriage: Part I", *Journal of Political Economy*, 1973, 81 (4).

[3] David De La Croix, F. Mariani, "From Polygyny to Serial Monogamy: A Unified Theory of Marriage Institutions", *Review of Economic Studies*, 2012, 82 (2).

[4] Shelly Lundberg, A. Pollak Robert, "The Evolving Role of Marriage: 1950-2010", *The Future of Children*, 2015, 25 (2).

F. Du et al., *Chinese People's Time Use and Their Quality of Life*,
https://doi.org/10.1007/978-981-99-5526-8_12

This chapter uses the 2017 Chinese Time Use Survey data from Inner Mongolia University to observe and analyze the relationship between couples in contemporary China in their time spent together and not together. The 2017 Chinese Time Use Survey data includes a total of 12,484 households, and after eliminating samples of those unmarried, widowed, and separated, and removing married samples younger than 20 years old and samples with missing important information such as gender and age, we matched a total of 8,987 couples based on the relationship between each family member and the "respondent".[5] In this chapter, all descriptive statistics and regression analyses are weighted by sampling weights.

Spending and Non-spending Time Together as a Couple

We divided the time spent with spouses into three categories: not spending time with the spouse (spouses participate in an activity separately, which include being alone and being with someone other than the spouse), spending time with the spouse and others (spouses participate in an activity together but with others participating at the same time), and spending time alone with the spouse (spouses participate in an activity at the same time without others participating).

Figure 12.1 reports the amount of time Chinese couples spent with and without their spouses of different ages in 2017. First, until age 70, couples' time spent together has always been longer than not together. Overall, couples spent 12.9 h per day not with their spouses, 3.0 h per day with spouses and others, and 8.1 h per day with their spouses. Second, as age increased, the time spent with spouses and others decreased, and the time spent just with spouses increased. For couples elder than 70 years old, more than half of the day was spent with their spouses. There is an old Chinese saying that goes "couples need the companion of each other when they grow old". In Fig. 12.1, although it is unclear what activities couples engage in together, the amount of time spent as companions to each other increases in old age. Finally, rural couples in China generally spend more time together than urban couples, and the reason for this is not that rural couples spend more time together alone, but that rural couples spend more time together with others.

Figure 12.2 reports the relationship between a couple's education levels and time spent with each other. The higher the education level, the more time spent not with spouses, which should be due to the fact that couples with higher education levels have independent jobs but couples with lower education levels are more likely to work together in household production and business or agricultural production activities; the higher the education level, the less time spent with their spouses, and the more time spent with others. If the time spent together, especially inclusive between the husband and wife, is positively correlated with the closeness of the relationship, and

[5] "Respondents" refers to the family members who were most likely to answer the questions at the time of the survey.

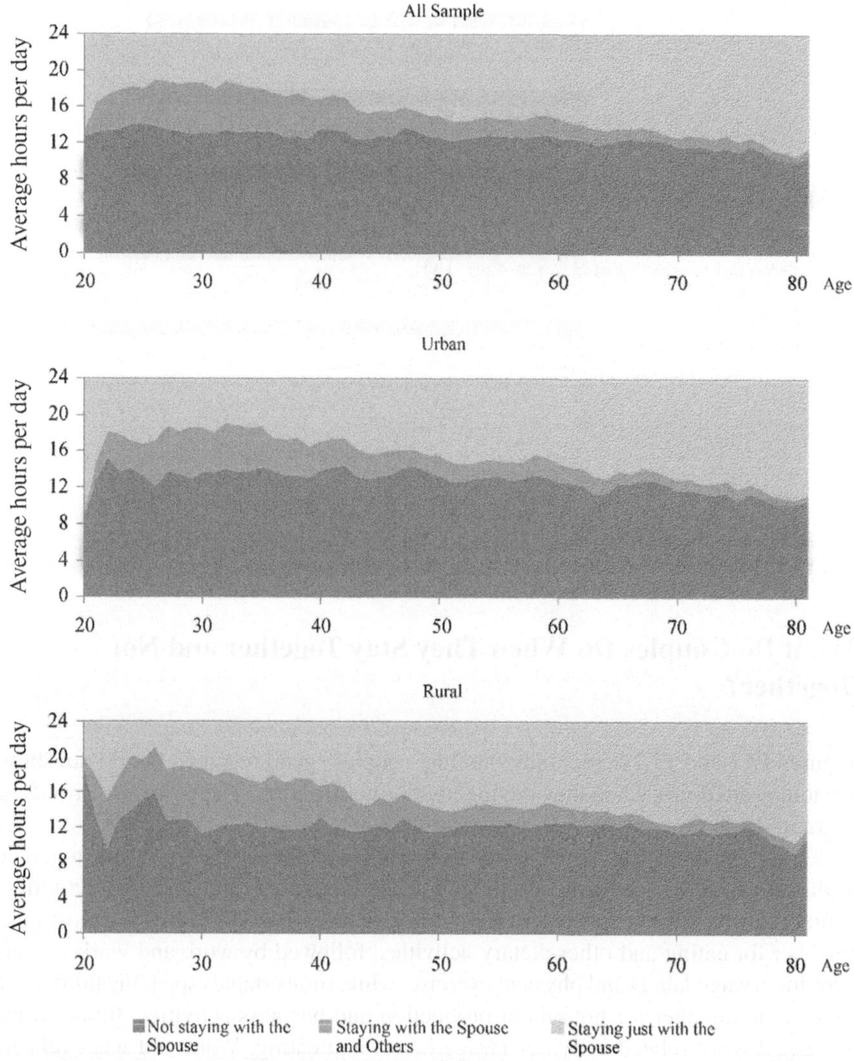

Fig. 12.1 Time spent with and without the spouse by age

without considering the activities couples engage in when they spend time together, it seems that the more educated couples are, the more indifferent the relationship is.

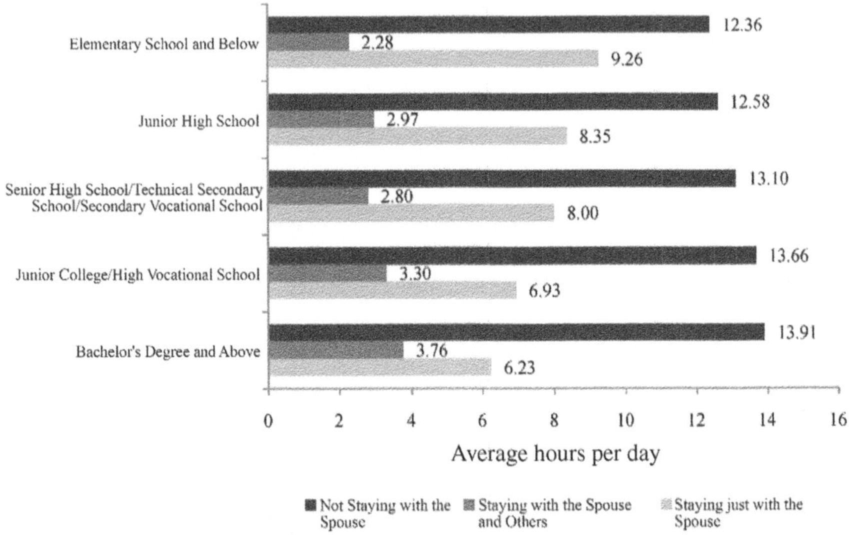

Fig. 12.2 Time spent with and without the spouse by education level

What Do Couples Do When They Stay Together and Not Together?

Figures 12.1 and 12.2 depict only the time couples spend together, but do not show what they are doing when they are together or not together. Therefore, we provide a more in-depth descriptive analysis in Fig. 12.3.

Figure 12.3 shows that both urban and rural couples spent the most time together within themselves for sleep, personal hygiene activities, and intimate activities, followed by recreation and leisure activities. Urban couples spent the third most time together for eating and other dietary activities, followed by work and work-related activities (wage labor) and physical exercise, while rural couples spent the third most time alone together for household production and business activities, followed by work and work-related activities (wage labor) and eating. Work and work-related activities (wage labor) were the most common activities that couples spent time on when they were not staying together. Urban couples spent the most time on work and work-related activities (wage labor), while rural couples spent the most time on sleep, personal hygiene activities, and intimate activities. Recreation and leisure were also activities that couples spent more time on when they were not staying together—about half of the recreation and leisure time was spent separately, indicating that Chinese couples' recreation and leisure activities were relatively independent. Comparisons between rural and urban areas show that the economic function of marriage is more significant in rural than in urban areas. On average, rural couples are more likely to engage in family production and operation activities together.

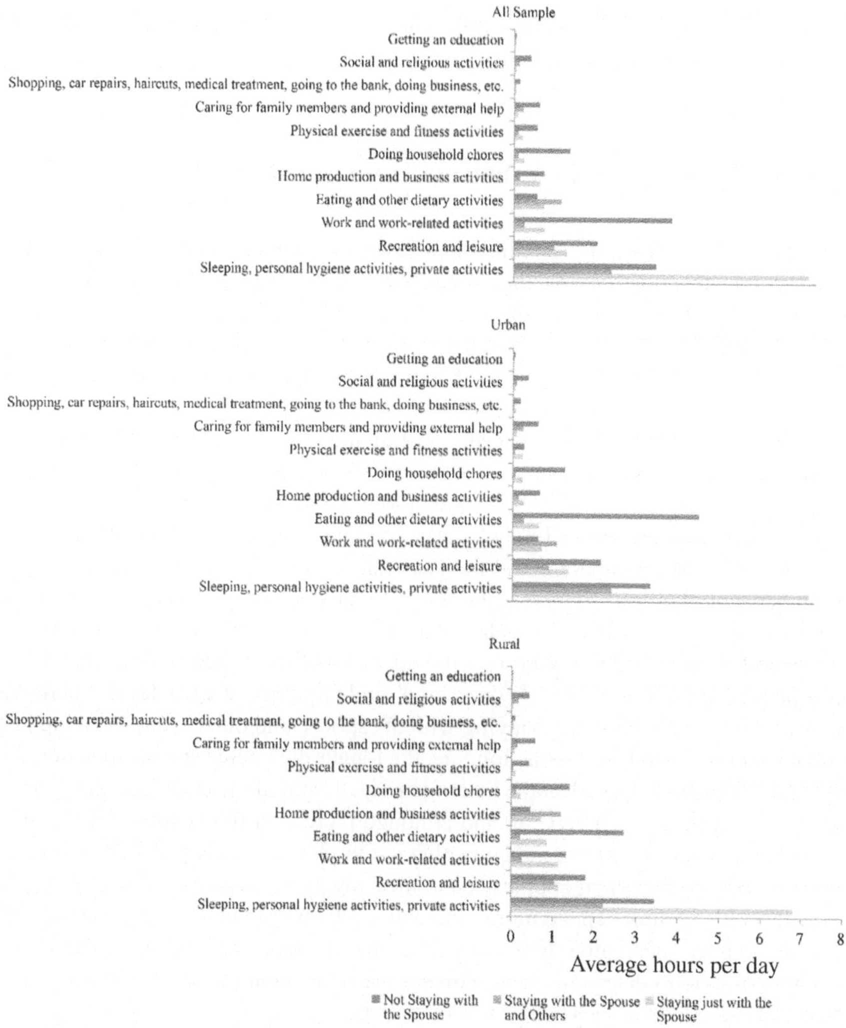

Fig. 12.3 Time use of residents and their spouses in different activities

Among a total of eleven major activities, some activities have low participation rates, such as getting educated. In Fig. 12.3, if someone did not participate in an activity, their time for that activity was zero. Then the mean was calculated between all sample points, which made differences in participation rates as well as would underestimate the amount of time activity participants spent on these activities. Therefore, in Table 12.1, we specifically report the average amount of time participants spent on that activity. Chinese spent less time on recreation and leisure when staying just with their spouses or with their spouses and others than when staying individually. Although the difference is small, they are also less likely to participate together than alone.

Spouses Time Spent Together and Life Satisfaction

As mentioned at the beginning of this chapter, we want to study Chinese couples' relationships by analyzing the time they spend together. Life satisfaction is an important indicator of couples' relationships. Each household member presented in the 2017 Chinese Time Use Survey was asked to rate life satisfaction (on a scale of 1–5): 1 for very satisfied and 5 for very dissatisfied. Figure 12.4 reports the relationship between the time couples spent and their life satisfaction. To simplify the analysis, we treated life satisfaction as a continuous variable and divided the time spent together into up to 150 intervals according to an interval every 10 min. Since the numbers of observations falling around 0 and 150 are much lower than the number of observations falling in the middle part, in Fig. 12.4 we weighted the number of observations in each interval with a nonparametric fit. The results show that, in general, the correlation between the time couples spent and life satisfaction is weak; when the time "not staying with the spouse" was less than 13 h, respondents' life satisfaction was largely independent of this type of time spent together. When it exceeded 13 h, respondents' satisfaction with life decreased[6] and remained at a low level. There is a positive relationship between "staying with the spouse and others" and "staying just with the spouse" and life satisfaction, i.e., the longer the couple spends together, the higher the life satisfaction. But the heterogeneity of "staying with spouse and others" increased significantly after 12 h, and although there is still a positive relationship with life satisfaction, which indicates that some people strongly dislike the presence of other people when couples spend time together, according to Fig. 12.1, we know that elder couples spend more time with each other than younger couples, and younger couples spend more time not with each other than older couples. Therefore, it is not possible to determine here whether the time spent together or not together affects life satisfaction or whether it is due to age.

In Fig. 12.3 and Table 12.1, we can see that couples spend the most time on sleep, personal hygiene, and intimate activities when being together; in the rural sample, couples also spend a lot of time together in productive activities. The former belongs to necessary physiological needs and the latter belongs to economic activity. The "enjoyment of life" is not common in these activities. Therefore, here we will specifically analyze the relationship between time use and life satisfaction of Chinese couples in recreation and leisure activities.

Figure 12.5 is similar to Fig. 12.4, except that the horizontal coordinate is replaced by the time spent on recreation and leisure activities. First, there is some correlation between time spent on recreation and leisure and life satisfaction, but the correlation is not high. Second, life satisfaction decreased more rapidly after each couple spent

[6] The larger the number, the lower the life satisfaction.

Table 12.1 Participation rates and time use of Chinese residents and their spouses in different activities

Activity		Not staying with the spouse		Staying with the spouse and others		Staying just with the spouse	
		Participation rate (%)	Average hours per day	Participation rate (%)	Average hours per day	Participation rate (%)	Average hours per day
Sleeping, personal hygiene activities, private activities	Urban	89.41	3.50	17.83	6.82	70.89	7.69
	Rural	85.73	3.90	17.85	6.95	66.87	7.96
Eating and other dietary activities	Urban	56.21	1.02	47.75	1.13	43.75	1.23
	Rural	42.32	1.04	51.87	1.13	43.86	1.23
Work and work-related activities	Urban	49.35	8.60	1.99	6.78	7.54	6.39
	Rural	32.39	8.12	2.12	5.59	10.55	6.30
Getting an education	Urban	0.99	3.46	0.07	1.71	0.09	2.93
	Rural	0.78	3.15	0.04	1.98	0.00	0.50
Home production and business activities	Urban	5.80	4.45	0.33	5.84	2.89	5.85
	Rural	26.06	4.91	2.18	6.31	14.50	6.11
Doing household chores	Urban	49.63	2.40	2.78	1.20	12.01	1.44
	Rural	50.65	2.70	2.40	2.65	10.66	1.48
Caring for family members and providing external help	Urban	16.26	3.57	4.64	2.83	2.39	2.65
	Rural	12.22	4.50	2.21	3.41	1.48	2.68

(continued)

Table 12.1 (continued)

Activity		Not staying with the spouse		Staying with the spouse and others		Staying just with the spouse	
		Participation rate (%)	Average hours per day	Participation rate (%)	Average hours per day	Participation rate (%)	Average hours per day
Shopping, car repairs, haircuts, medical treatment, going to the bank, doing business, etc.	Urban	10.01	1.57	0.55	2.13	2.08	1.78
	Rural	3.37	2.17	0.41	1.84	1.23	2.74
Physical exercise and fitness activities	Urban	26.74	2.25	4.34	1.58	9.90	1.86
	Rural	17.17	2.36	1.37	1.24	4.00	1.77
Recreation and leisure	Urban	58.32	3.44	18.87	2.36	34.14	2.94
	Rural	50.55	3.44	23.48	2.47	32.79	2.72
Social and religious activities	Urban	12.33	2.82	1.98	1.84	1.96	1.43
	Rural	13.19	3.04	3.47	2.45	1.63	1.44

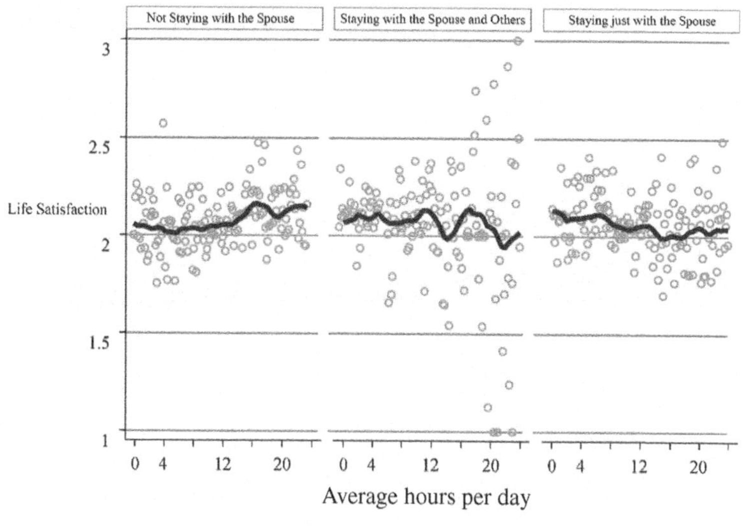

Fig. 12.4 Relationship between time spent with the spouse and life satisfaction. *Note* Life satisfaction: 1—very satisfied, 2—satisfied, 3—average, 4—dissatisfied, 5—very dissatisfied, the same below

more than 11 h on recreation and leisure activities; in both the "staying with spouse and others" and "staying just with spouse" graphs, there is an extreme value of very low satisfaction, but removing the extremes or not has no significant effect on the results: the amount of time couples spend together for recreation is not significantly related to life satisfaction.

Figure 12.5 raises the question: why is the amount of time spent on recreation and leisure when couples stay together so weakly correlated with life satisfaction? Perhaps the question is not about quantity—the amount of time couples spent together for recreation and leisure—but about quality—how they do it, and whether these recreational activities actually lead to spiritual enjoyment or satisfaction? Therefore, in the next section, we will further analyze what Chinese couples do during their recreation and leisure time.

What Do Couples Do During Recreation and Leisure?

In this subsection, we analyze the time arrangement of Chinese couples for recreation and leisure activities. Figure 12.6 reports the time use of Chinese residents and their spouses on different recreation and leisure activities. Overall, watching TV and resting, hobbies, games and recreational activities are the two types of recreational and leisure activities that cost the most time, far exceeding the time spent on other activities. When couples spent time together (both within themselves and with others), the activity that consumed the most time was watching TV, followed

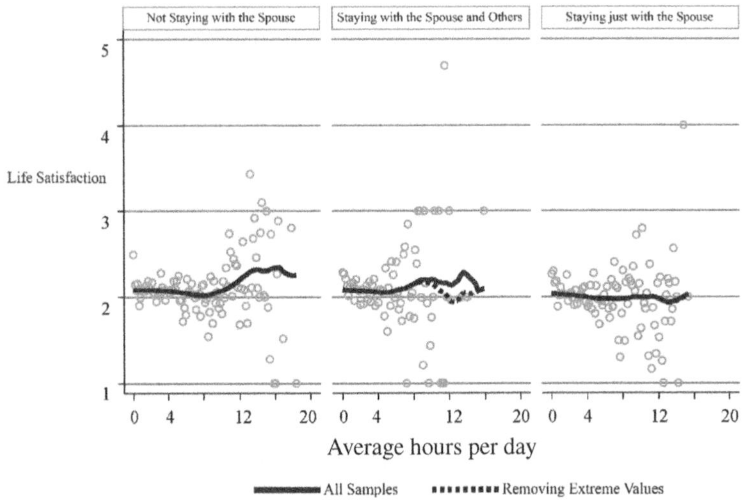

Fig. 12.5 Time spent with the spouse on recreation and leisure activities and life satisfaction. *Note* Life satisfaction: 1—very satisfied, 2—satisfied, 3—average, 4—dissatisfied, 5—very dissatisfied, the same below

by resting, hobbies, games, and recreational activities. The most time spent when couples were not staying together was on rest, hobbies, games and recreational leisure, followed by watching TV. In addition, e-reading was also a very important recreation and leisure activity for couples when they were not staying together.

Table 12.2 reports the participation rates of couples in different recreation and leisure activities and the average time spent on each activity. First of all, watching TV and resting, hobby, games and recreation activities were the two activities with the highest participation rates: about 30% of urban couples spent nearly 3 h per day on these two activities when they were not staying together, and around 30% of urban couples also spent approximately 3 h per day watching TV when they were living alone together; the situation was similar for rural couples as for urban couples. Among other recreational activities, except for cell phone reading and activities using other media, the participation rate of other recreational activities was very low. They spent more time on individual activities, such as "outings, movies, and shows".

Both Fig. 12.6 and Table 12.2 show that watching TV and resting, hobbies, games and recreation activities were the two most important forms of recreation and leisure for Chinese couples. However, it is worth noting that these are the two least costly recreation and leisure activities. In Fig. 12.7, we focus on the heterogeneity of these two activities in terms of educational attainment. First, the time spent watching TV with spouse and others was about 20 min per day and was not significantly related to education level. Second, as education level increased, the average time spent watching TV per day decreased, whether staying with spouses or not. Finally, Chinese residents' "resting, hobbies, games, and recreational activities" were more of an individual activity and were rarely done with their spouses, and this was true

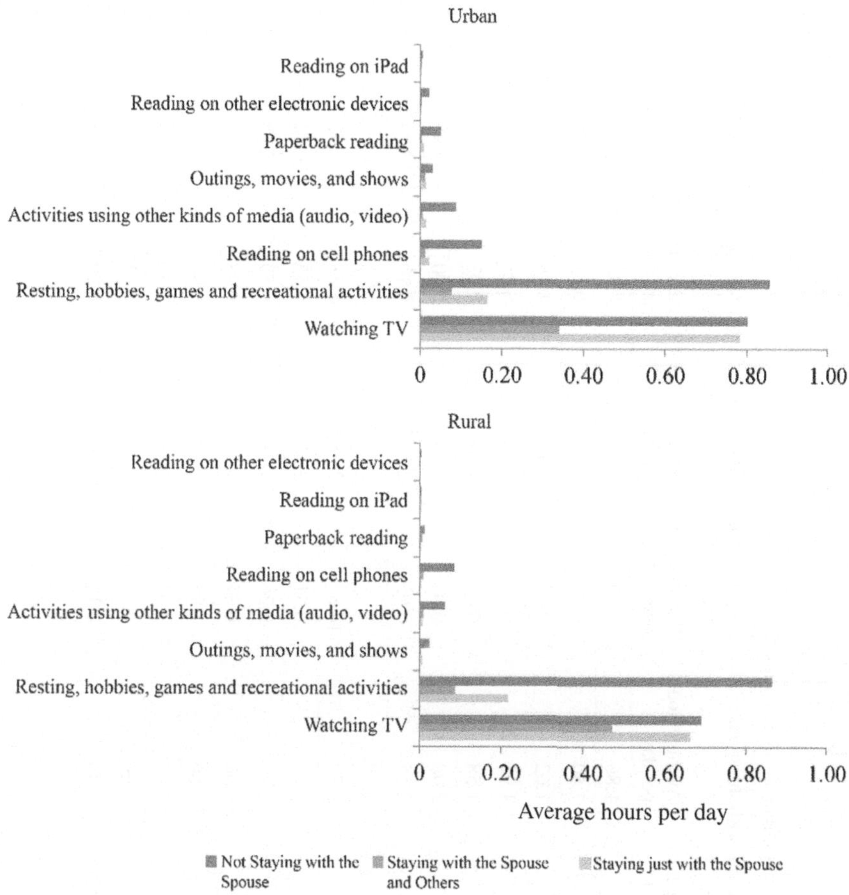

Fig. 12.6 Couple's time use patterns on different recreation and leisure activities

across education levels. As education levels increased, couples spent less time on this activity when they are not living together.

In terms of activity duration, "resting, hobbies, games and recreational activities" are among the two most important forms of recreation and leisure for Chinese residents. Table 12.3 shows that the highest participation rate in this category is resting, followed by card and board games (in the Chinese context, chess and tile activities largely refer to Mahjong). It is worth noting that some activities had relatively low participation rates, but participants spent a lot of time on them. For example, in the urban samples, although participation rates for playing computer games with spouses and others were low, people spent about 6 h per day on it. In addition, if we add together time on mobile games, computer games, and tabletop games (collectively referred to as video games), the participation rate of urban couples when they

Table 12.2 Participation rate and time use of couples in different recreation activities

Activity		Not staying with the spouse		Staying with the spouse and others		Staying just with the spouse	
		Participation rate (%)	Average hours per day	Participation rate (%)	Average hours per day	Participation rate (%)	Average hours per day
Paperback reading	Urban	2.77	1.86	0.20	1.42	0.38	2.00
	Rural	0.71	1.50	0.19	2.69	0.13	0.59
Reading on cell phones	Urban	9.35	1.62	0.73	1.49	1.16	1.83
	Rural	4.34	1.95	0.33	2.06	0.25	1.14
Reading on iPad	Urban	0.28	1.58	0.01	1.19	0.02	1.29
	Rural	0.05	1.98	0.03	0.33	0.00	4.98
Reading on other electronic devices	Urban	0.84	2.55	0.05	2.50	0.10	3.24
	Rural	0.21	1.59				
Watching TV	Urban	29.05	2.76	14.87	2.28	28.78	2.72
	Rural	25.42	2.72	20.31	2.32	27.55	2.41
Activities using other kinds of media (audio, video)	Urban	3.85	2.27	0.26	1.78	0.59	2.08
	Rural	2.13	2.90	0.37	1.96	0.28	1.71
Resting, hobbies, games and recreational activities	Urban	29.94	2.86	3.93	1.93	6.98	2.35
	Rural	28.29	3.05	3.64	2.38	7.50	2.89
Outings, movies, and shows	Urban	0.78	3.69	0.29	3.66	0.43	2.82
	Rural	0.68	3.46	0.11	2.50	0.20	2.48

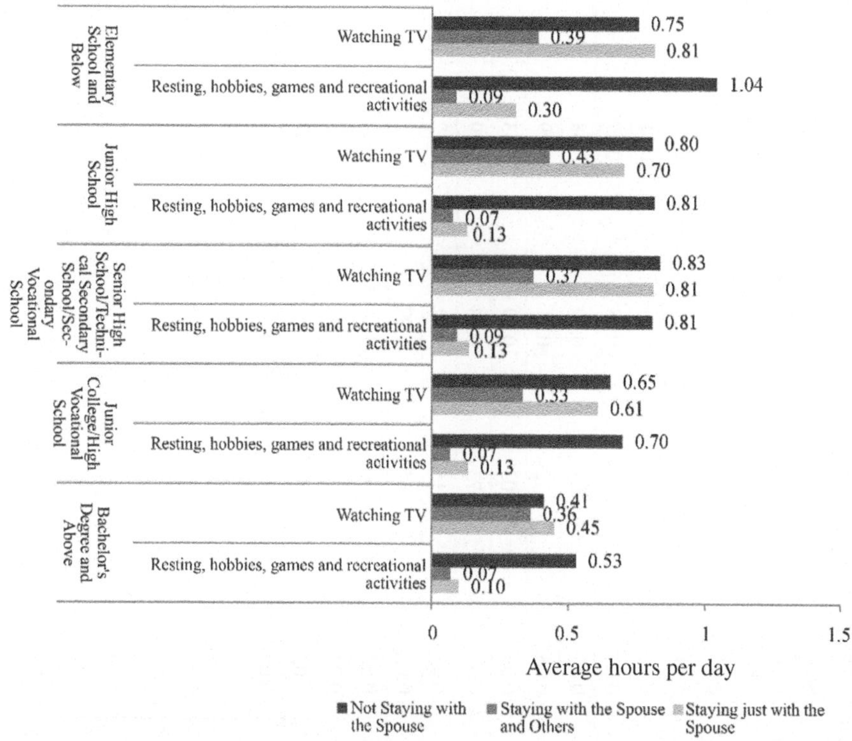

Fig. 12.7 Time spent on the two main recreation and leisure activities by couples with different education levels

are not staying together will be 3.36%,[7] and the average daily time spent will be 2.85 h; the participation rate of rural couples when they are not staying together will be 1.32% and the average daily time spent will be 2.57 h; although couples rarely play games when they are staying together (both within themselves and with others), they spend a lot of time once they play, or even more. This shows that the population of video games may not be large, but the impact of video games on the daily life of these "players" is not small in terms of time use.

Does Time Spent with the Spouse Affect Life Satisfaction?

We analyzed the amount of time couples spend together and not together on different activities, focusing on recreation and leisure activities because these activities can be considered more of a "life enjoyment" and are more likely to reflect the non-economic

[7] This participation rate is lower than the sum of these activities in Table 12.3 because some people participate in two or more activities at the same time.

Table 12.3 Couples' participation rates and time spent on resting, hobbies, games, and recreation activities

Activity		Not staying with the spouse		Staying with the spouse and others		Staying just with the spouse	
		Participation rate (%)	Average hours per day	Participation rate (%)	Average hours per day	Participation rate (%)	Average hours per day
Resting	Urban	19.39	2.18	2.89	1.72	5.68	2.28
	Rural	21.32	2.60	3.44	2.39	7.02	2.93
Smoking	Urban	0.31	0.45			0.04	0.61
	Rural	0.37	0.82	0.02	0.17	0.08	0.27
Card and board games	Urban	4.63	3.99	0.25	2.61	0.29	3.38
	Rural	3.35	4.08	0.06	4.12	0.01	2.19
Mobile games	Urban	1.66	2.11	0.09	3.03	0.19	1.43
	Rural	0.60	2.51	0.01	1.73	0.08	1.29
Playing mobile games	Urban	0.42	2.02	0.05	1.15	0.02	1.22
	Rural	0.41	2.03	0.03	1.85	0.00	
Computer games	Urban	0.89	3.90	0.02	6.00	0.16	3.64
	Rural	0.19	2.40	0.00		0.00	
Playing online games	Urban	0.49	3.54	0.02	3.25	0.02	3.53
	Rural	0.23	2.55	0.00		0.00	

(continued)

Table 12.3 (continued)

Activity		Not staying with the spouse		Staying with the spouse and others		Staying just with the spouse	
		Participation rate (%)	Average hours per day	Participation rate (%)	Average hours per day	Participation rate (%)	Average hours per day
Playing tabletop games	Urban	0.01	4.20	0.00		0.00	
	Rural	0.00		0.00		0.00	
Singing	Urban	0.16	2.58	0.01	1.98	0.01	1.88
	Rural	0.01	2.16	0.00		0.00	
Philately and other collecting activities	Urban	0.02	3.29	0.00		0.00	
	Rural	0.00	3.98	0.00		0.00	
Literature and art activities	Urban	0.49	3.43	0.01	3.31	0.04	3.01
	Rural	0.10	2.57	0.00		0.00	
Other hobbies	Urban	4.12	2.82	0.41	1.84		
	Rural	3.59	3.40	0.10	1.51	0.38	2.20
Related transportation activities	Urban	1.15	0.75	0.13	0.30	0.22	0.69
	Rural	0.83	0.60	0.02	0.39	0.22	0.44

aspects of the marital relationship. Therefore, based on the nature of the activities and whether they require or elicit positive interactions from the participants, we grouped the activities into the following five categories (see Annexed Table 12.6 at the end of this chapter for a detailed breakdown): (1) physiological needs (e.g., sleeping and eating); (2) economic activities (wage labor and household production activities); (3) domestic production (e.g., doing housework, tutoring children's homework, etc.); (4) active interactions (e.g., going on trips and playing with children); and (5) passive interactions (e.g., watching TV, playing computer games, etc.).

The first part of Table 12.4 reports the participation rates of urban and rural couples in the five major activities and the average length spent on each activity. The table shows that physiological needs and economic activities occupy most of the time in daily life; the participation rates and time spent on active interaction activities are generally less than those on passive interaction activities; and the interactive activities with a spouse (both within themselves and with others) are much less than without a spouse. The second part of Table 12.4 studies Chinese couples' participation rates in the five major activities and the average amount of time spent by gender. The results show that husbands spend more time participating in economic activities alone while wives in household production, which is consistent with the traditional labor division within the family. Otherwise, there was little difference in the time use of couples in the five major categories of activities with and without their spouses. There is little difference between husbands and wives in terms of participation rates and time use for active and passive interaction activities: both are more likely to engage in passive activities than active activities, and more likely to engage in them separately than together.

Effective communication and spiritual companionship between couples are more likely to be achieved when couples spend time together. So the amount of time spent together and the activities couples engage in when they are together are strongly related to subjective well-being.[8] Figures 12.4 and 12.5 show that the amount of time couples spend together is related to life satisfaction, but the relationship is not strong. Here we further use regression analysis to examine the relationship between the time couples spend together and life satisfaction. The results are shown in Table 12.5.

For the life satisfaction variable, larger values indicate greater dissatisfaction with life. So column (1) indicates that the longer the couple spends together (with or without other people present), the higher the life satisfaction. Similar results were obtained by Flood and Genadek's study of time spent together and not together for couples in the U.S.[9] Since there are only 24 h in a day, adding couples' non-together time to the regression analysis would lead to full multi-collinearity. So it was not included in the regression model. Column (2) shows that recreation and leisure time

[8] Melisa A. Milkie, P. Peltola, "Playing All the Roles: Gender and the Work-family Balancing Act", *Journal of Marriage & Family*, 1999, 61 (2); Kerry J. Daly, "Deconstructing Family Time: From Ideology to Lived Experience", *Journal of Marriage & Family*, 2001, 63 (2); Constance T. Gager, Laura Sanchez, "Two as One? Couples' Perceptions of Time Spent Together, Marital Quality, and the Risk of Divorce", *Journal of Family Issues*, 2003, 24 (1).

[9] Sarah M. Flood, Katie R. Genadek, "Time for Each Other: Work and Family Constraints Among Couples", *Journal of Marriage and Family*, 2016, 78 (1).

Table 12.4 Chinese couples' participation rate and time use in the five major categories of activities

Activity		Not staying with the spouse		Staying with the spouse and others		Staying just with the spouse	
		Participation rate (%)	Average hours per day	Participation rate (%)	Average hours per day	Participation rate (%)	Average hours per day
By urban and rural areas							
Physiological needs	Urban	92.91	3.92	50.39	3.48	75.68	7.91
	Rural	88.42	4.25	53.59	3.55	73.15	8.04
Economic activities	Urban	54.30	8.29	2.30	6.70	10.20	6.38
	Rural	55.19	7.08	4.29	5.96	23.72	6.54
Home production	Urban	56.07	3.20	6.30	2.22	14.58	1.80
	Rural	54.49	3.43	4.06	3.01	12.47	1.78
Active interactions	Urban	41.91	3.10	8.65	1.94	12.98	1.97
	Rural	34.87	3.20	5.78	2.29	6.49	1.88
Passive interactions	Urban	56.65	3.25	18.43	2.30	33.76	2.90
	Rural	49.14	3.25	23.39	2.47	32.65	2.70
By gender							
Physiological needs	Husband	91.15	3.96	51.00	3.46	75.35	7.96
	Wife	90.98	4.20	52.45	3.56	73.88	7.96

(continued)

Table 12.4 (continued)

Activity		Not staying with the spouse		Staying with the spouse and others		Staying just with the spouse	
		Participation rate (%)	Average hours per day	Participation rate (%)	Average hours per day	Participation rate (%)	Average hours per day
Economic activities	Husband	63.95	8.23	3.03	6.27	15.78	6.58
	Wife	44.79	7.11	3.22	6.30	15.72	6.36
Home production	Husband	32.54	2.22	4.28	2.55	13.05	1.80
	Wife	79.75	3.76	6.55	2.41	14.41	1.79
Active interactions	Husband	38.16	3.26	7.74	2.11	10.60	1.94
	Wife	39.93	3.01	7.18	1.98	10.02	1.95
Passive interactions	Husband	56.10	3.31	21.26	2.45	33.60	2.90
	Wife	50.87	3.18	19.63	2.30	32.98	2.74

Table 12.5 Relationship between life satisfaction and time spent together as a couple

	(1)	(2)	(3)	(4)	(5)	(6)	(7)	(8)	(9)
Time spent with the spouse and others (hours)	−0.005* (0.003)								
Time spent alone with the spouse (hours)	−0.004** (0.002)								
Recreation and leisure time spent not with the spouse (hours)		0.003 (0.004)							
Recreation and leisure time spent with the spouse and others (hours)		−0.016** (0.007)							
Recreational and leisure time spent with the spouse alone (hours)		−0.007 (0.005)							
Time spent actively interacting without spending time with the spouse (hours)			−0.013*** (0.004)						−0.014*** (0.005)
Active interaction time spent with spouse and others (hours)				0.006 (0.017)					0.007 (0.017)

(continued)

Table 12.5 (continued)

	(1)	(2)	(3)	(4)	(5)	(6)	(7)	(8)	(9)
Active interaction time spent with spouse alone (hours)					−0.012 (0.012)				−0.015 (0.012)
Time spent in passive interaction without spending time with spouse (hours)						0.005 (0.004)			0.002 (0.004)
Passive interactions spent with spouse and others (hours)							−0.017** (0.007)		−0.020*** (0.008)
Passive interactions with spouse alone (hours)								−0.005 (0.005)	−0.008 (0.005)
Sample size	17924	17924	17924	17924	17924	17924	17924	17924	17924
R^2	0.047	0.047	0.047	0.046	0.046	0.047	0.047	0.046	0.049

Note The dependent variable is the life satisfaction: 1—very satisfied; 2—satisfied; 3—fair; 4—dissatisfied; 5—very dissatisfied. The numbers in parentheses are standard errors, and standard errors are clustered at the household level. ***, **, and * indicate that the estimated coefficients passed significance tests at the 1, 5, and 10% levels, respectively. All regressions control for gender, household registration, urban-rural classification of residence, age and its squared term, education level, employment status, income level, and dummy variables indicating missing income variables and province fixed effects.

spent together by couples increases life satisfaction, but it is only statistically significant when couples spend time with other people (generally family members and especially children). From columns (3) to (8), we place the two types of interactions defined in this section into regression models for each of the three couple coexistence situations and find that active interactions with others rather than the spouse and passive interactions with the spouse and others significantly increase life satisfaction; active and passive interactions with the spouse alone have similar effects, but are not statistically significant. This result is slightly surprising, but space limitations prevent this chapter from digging further into the reasons and implications. Column (9) places the six time use situations for the two interaction styles grouped according to the three situations where couples stay together in the regression model. The regression results are essentially the same as those in columns (3) through (8), except for a slight change in the absolute value of the coefficients.

Summary

This chapter examines Chinese couples' time together. The main findings are: (1) Chinese couples spend a lot of time with each other only when they are old; (2) the higher the education level, the shorter the time couples spend alone; (3) Chinese couples' recreation and leisure when they spend time together is mainly watching TV, and when they do not spend time together is "resting, hobbies, games and recreation activities"; (4) The participation rate of interaction between couples, especially active interaction, is relatively low and the amount of time is relatively low; and (5) on average, the correlation between time spent together and life satisfaction is weak, which may be related to the fact that the activities performed by couples when they spend time together are not active and interesting.

Chinese couples or families are more of a productive unit, with economic activities and household production taking up most of the time except for physiological needs. Recreation and leisure are dominated by watching TV and resting. Couples are less interactive with each other, and the happiness that couples get when they spend time alone is lower than the happiness when they spend time with others. Therefore, the current situation in Chinese marital relationships is that the economic function is more important than the soul mate. Life is dull and unexciting. Although it is said that "a simple life is a true life", "simple" does not exclude "wonderful" daily life.

Annexed Table 12.6 Classification of activity types based on the interaction between couples

Classification	Activity
1 Physiological needs	01: Sleeping, personal hygiene activities and intimate activities
	0201: Eating
2 Economic activities	03: Work and work-related activities (wage labor)
	05: Home production
3 Home production	0401–0405: Various formal education
	0601–0604, 0606, 0688, 0699: Housework
	070101–070103, 070105, 070107–070109, 070301–070303, 070305, 070307–070399: Caring for minors
	0702: Caring for adult family members
	080101, 080199: Shopping and transportation activities
	080201-080205, 080299: Online shopping activities and related transportation activities
	0803: Repairing automobiles, electrical appliances, etc.
	0805: Medical treatment
	0806: Banking
	0807: Finding home management, training, education and agency
	0808: Other businesses
4 Active interactions	0202: Other dietary activities
	0406: Non-formal education
	0605: Keeping pets
	0607: Arrangement of family affairs
	070104, 070106, 070304, 070306: Reading with children and playing with children
	0705: Unpaid housework help to other families
	0706: Participation in community service and public welfare activities
	080102: Shopping
	080206: Viewing
	0804: Haircutting, beauty care, bathing, health care
	09: Physical exercise and fitness activities
	100709–100799: Playing, various activities such as literature and art, and transportation
	1008: Outings, movies and shows
	1101: Face-to-face social interactions
	1103: Religious activities
5 Passive interactions	1001–1004: Reading
	1005: Watching TV
	1006: Other activities using media
	100701–100708: Resting and games
	1102: Non-face-to-face social interactions

Chapter 13
Impact of Phones on Residents' Time Use

The revolution of information technology has dramatically changed the way of production and living. Especially since the last decade, the popularity of cell phones has made the Internet accessible to everyone. Cell phones are also becoming increasingly functional, encompassing all aspects of calling, chatting, searching, reading, video, music, payment, and medical care, as people move from real daily life to an online life centered on digital information technology.

In developing countries, there is a digital divide due to inequality in accessibility, application, and innovation of information technology among residents. Along with changes in the online media environment and innovations in Internet Technology (IT), the digital divide has led to differences in people's participation, habits, and information possession, leading to social stratification.[1] The difference in information accessibility is called the First Digital Divide, and the difference in application and identification is called the Second Digital Divide. As cell phones are gaining popularity in urban and rural areas at an alarming rate, this innovation of information technology plays a crucial role in bridging the digital divide between countries, regions, industries, enterprises, and communities. It has become essential for the Information-Proletariat to improve their quality of life.[2] At present, China's communication infrastructure has been improved, and the First Digital Divide has been basically bridged. But in the information explosion era, people with poor information application and identification ability cannot obtain accurate and practical information. There is a large Second Digital Divide.[3] With the development of cell phones, people's time allocation has started to change significantly, and time is a scarce

[1] Li Yan, Li Qiu, "From Class Division in Online Communication to Cultural Barriers in the Age of We Media—The Evolution and Impact of the Development Pattern of Digital Divide", *Journalism Lover*, 2014 (6).

[2] BBC, "Mobile Growth 'Fastest in Africa'", http://news.bbc.co.uk/2/hi/business/4331863.stm, 2005.

[3] Zhuqing Xu, Fengtian Zheng, Jie Chen, "The 'Digital Divide' or the 'Information Dividend'? Effective Supply of Information and Farmers' Selling Prices—An Empirical Study from a Micro Perspective", *China Economic Quarterly*, 2013 (4).

F. Du et al., *Chinese People's Time Use and Their Quality of Life*,
https://doi.org/10.1007/978-981-99-5526-8_13

resource, so the efficiency of time allocation and application is related to workers' utility and welfare level.[4]

This chapter uses data from the 2017 Chinese Time Use Survey to discuss the problems mentioned above. First, it introduces the current Chinese residents' phone ownership, usage, the average length of time spent using phones, and what activities they use them for. Then, it analyzes the impact of socioeconomic factors such as age, education, urban and rural division, gender, employment status, and income on whether or not to use phones, the length of use, and the usage of phones. Then it explores whether the digital divide exists in China currently. Finally, it analyzes the impact of cell phones on the time allocation of residents. This section shows which activities and time periods are crowded out by phones. The result helps to study the impact of cell phone use on the quality of life of Chinese residents.

Overview of Residents' Phone Use

This section focuses on the phone ownership rate of Chinese residents, as well as the phone use of people with different income, occupation and education levels, with data from the 2017 Chinese Time Use Survey (CTUS) and the 2017 China Household Finance Survey (CHFS). Residents in the age group of 10–80 years old were selected as the study population, with a total sample size of 26,251, including 15,466 urban samples (58.9%) and 10,785 rural samples (41.1%). Regarding gender, 13,226 of them were male, accounting for 50.4%; 13,025 were female, accounting for 49.6%.

Figure 13.1a shows the proportion of all household owners in the CHFS sample who owned a phone. It can be seen that the proportion of Chinese residents' phone ownership reached 95.2%, of which 63.0% owned a cell phone, 32.3% owned a non-cell phone, and only 4.8% did not own a phone.

Figure 13.1b shows the use of cell phones by the full sample of residents on the day being surveyed. It can be seen that 23.4% of the sample used cell phones on the day of the survey. Possible reasons for the smaller proportion of cell phone use than cell phone ownership include: (1) farmers did not carry their cell phones for labor on the survey day; (2) workers did not have time to use their cell phones in the course of their work due to the heavy tasks they undertook; (3) a significant portion of the older population owned cell phones but did not know how to use them due to reasons like lower literacy levels; (4) although respondents used their cell phones several times during the day, the length of each use was less than 10 min, so they were not counted; (5) residents use cell phones during work and transportation, but they did not report it.

Figure 13.2 shows the phone usage rate of different income groups. The income variable is measured according to the quintile of per capita household income in each province, which avoids the impact of income differences in provinces. The phone

[4] Floro, M. S., "Economic Restructuring, Gender and the Allocation of Time", *World Development*, 1995, 23(11).

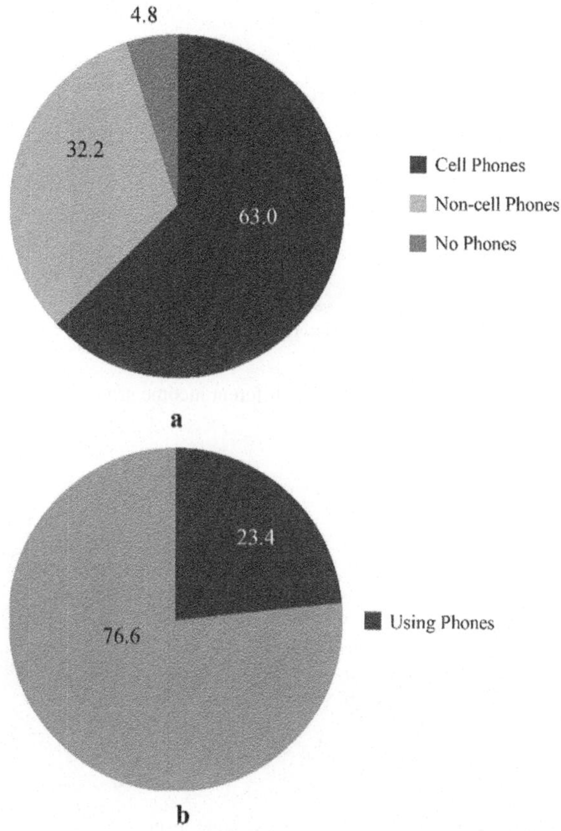

Fig. 13.1 **a** Proportion of Chinese residents owning phones (%). **b** Proportion of Chinese residents using cell phones (%)

usage rate and income are positively correlated. The usage rate of phones increases with income. The phone usage rate of high-income people is 2.4 times higher than that of low-income people.

From Fig. 13.3, it can be seen that there is a positive correlation between the phone usage rate and the residents' education level. The phone usage rate increased with education level. Among them, the phone usage rate of residents with a bachelor's degree or above is 20.2 times higher than that of the unschooled.

As seen from Fig. 13.4, the phone usage rate of residents engaged in agriculture, forestry, animal husbandry, and fishery production was the lowest at 14.0%, while the phone usage rate of professional and technical personnel was the highest at 39.5%. The difference between other occupations is not significant.

As seen from Fig. 13.5, the most common activities of Chinese residents when using cell phones were e-reading, phone socializing, watching or listening, and playing phone games. People reading on phones took up the largest proportion of 63.9%, followed by watching and listening on phones, which was 31.8%, and then by playing phone games, which was the smallest at only 6.2%.

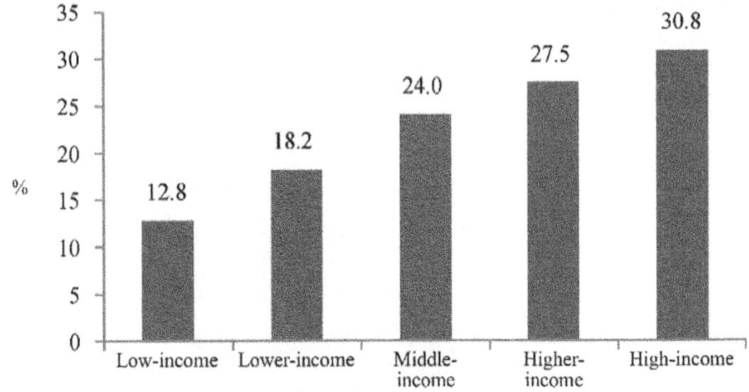

Fig. 13.2 Phone usage rate of different income groups

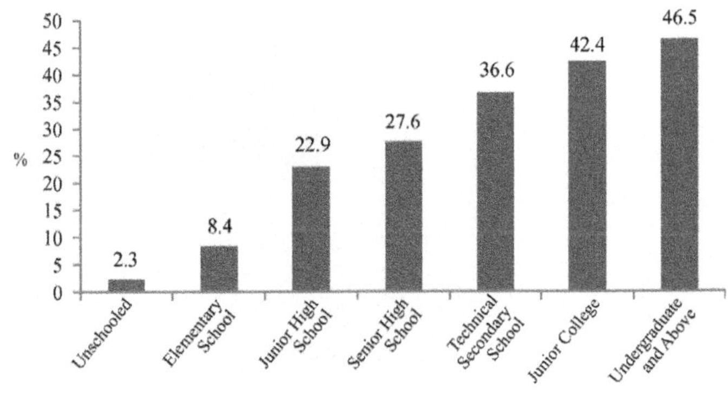

Fig. 13.3 Phone usage rate by education level

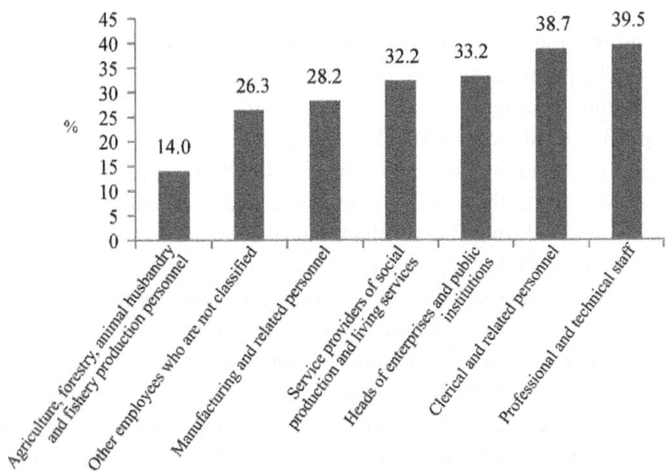

Fig. 13.4 Phone usage rate by occupation

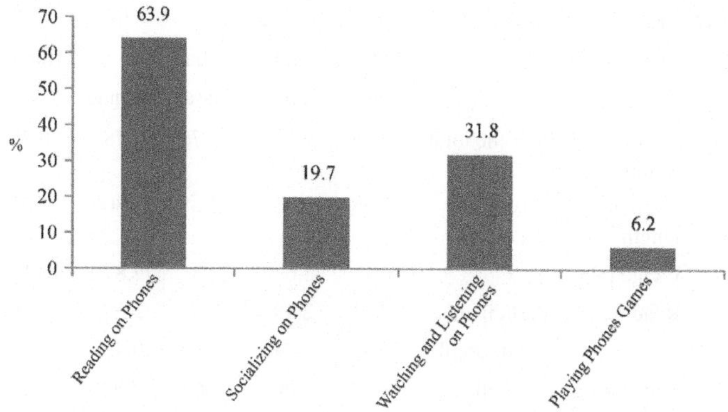

Fig. 13.5 Phone usage rate by application

The Digital Divide

This section analyzes in detail the differences in phone usage by age, education, employment status, urban and rural division, gender, marital status and income. Firstly, a descriptive statistical analysis of phone usage is conducted, followed by a regression analysis of phone hours and usage rates. Then, it further analyzes the participation rates of various phone uses among different groups of people.

Overall Situation

From Table 13.1, it can be seen that the average length of phone use in the total sample did not exceed 1 h, both nationwide and in urban and rural areas. But the average length of participants was higher than 2.5 h. In terms of phone usage rates and usage purposes, the usage rates were higher in urban areas than in rural areas, and the average length of time spent reading on phones was the longest among the four purposes. The average length of time spent reading by rural residents was lower than that of urban residents. The differences in the average length of time spent by participants in each of the other purposes are not significant.

Table 13.2 reports the regression results of the length of phone use and usage rate. It can be seen that the average length of cell phone use and usage rate of residents aged 19–30 years old had increased compared with those aged 10–18 years old, with the longest length and the highest usage rate being among residents aged 19–22 years old. This age group coincides with college students, who have more time and are more likely to accept and master new things. In terms of education level, the time length and usage rate of phones increased with education level compared to those who had not attended school. There is no significant effect of gender on the use of

Table 13.1 Descriptive statistics of phone usage. Unit: hours/day

Population			National total		Urban		Rural	
			Male	Female	Male	Female	Male	Female
General information	Average length of the total sample		0.65	0.61	0.76	0.78	0.48	0.38
	Average participants length		2.68	2.72	2.68	2.80	2.67	2.50
	Usage rate (%)		24.1	22.6	28.3	27.8	18.1	15.3
Average participation length by usage	Reading	Participants	2.41	2.49	2.42	2.58	2.40	2.21
		Total sample	0.38	0.34	0.46	0.45	0.25	0.19
	Socializing	Participants	2.03	2.00	2.05	2.02	1.98	1.93
		Total sample	0.09	0.09	0.10	0.11	0.08	0.05
	Watching and listening	Participants	2.00	2.13	2.03	2.06	1.93	2.30
		Total sample	0.13	0.17	0.15	0.19	0.11	0.13
	Playing games	Participants	2.14	1.72	2.07	1.80	2.27	1.37
		Total sample	0.05	0.01	0.05	0.02	0.04	0.01

cell phones. Unmarried residents use phones more than married. Urban residents use phones more than rural residents in length and usage rate.

It can be seen that with the increase in income, the average length and usage rate also grew, but the increase is small. Different brands of cell phones satisfy all kinds of customers with low-, medium- and high-grade needs. There are alternatives for phones of different price levels, but there is no difference in usage. Therefore, income is no longer the main factor affecting phone usage.

From the above findings, it can be seen that the use of cell phones and information application of Chinese residents are influenced to some extent by urban and rural division, education level, employment status and marital status. There are some differences in the usage rate and length of phones among different groups of people. Therefore, although cell phones have effectively improved the convenience in using information and communication, there is still a certain degree of digital divide among different groups of people in China.

Analysis of Phone Usage

In this sub-section, phone usage is divided into four categories: reading, socializing, watching and listening, and playing games on phones. The differences in the usage rates of phones are explored by age, urban and rural division, gender and employment status.

Table 13.2 Regression results of phone usage length and usage rate

Variables		(1) Average length	(2) Average participants length	(3) Used or not
Age (reference group: 10–18)	19–22	0.459** (2.29)	0.358 (1.06)	0.096** (2.43)
	23–30	0.046 (0.20)	−0.113 (−0.31)	0.052 (1.19)
	31–40	−0.298 (−1.29)	−0.403 (−1.06)	−0.015 (−0.35)
	41–50	−0.525** (−2.29)	−0.545 (−1.44)	−0.097** (−2.20)
	51–60	−0.747*** (−3.26)	−0.506 (−1.32)	−0.201*** (−4.58)
	61–70	−0.857*** (−3.73)	−0.697* (−1.75)	−0.237*** (−5.40)
	71–80	−0.934*** (−4.06)	−0.485 (1.07)	−0.266*** (−6.03)
Education level (reference group: unschooled)	Elementary school	0.068*** (3.76)	−0.112 (−0.30)	0.023*** (4.74)
	Junior high school	0.279*** (11.47)	−0.108 (−0.30)	0.107*** (17.03)
	Senior high school	0.327*** (9.54)	−0.142 (−0.39)	0.135*** (15.03)
	Technical secondary school	0.440*** (7.56)	−0.018 (−0.05)	0.165*** (11.63)
	Junior college	0.509*** (9.37)	−0.061 (−0.17)	0.194*** (13.54)
	Undergraduate and above	0.513*** (8.83)	−0.085 (−0.23)	0.194*** (13.54)
Marital status (unmarried = 1)		0.371*** (5.34)	0.674** (4.73)	0.037*** (2.59)
Gender (male = 1)		−0.015 (−0.74)	0.070 (1.01)	−0.009* (−1.70)
Urban and rural (rural = 1)		−0.104*** (−4.96)	0.176* (1.84)	−0.058*** (−11.07)
Employment status (reference group: unemployed)	Students	−0.345* (−2.12)	−0.966*** (−3.74)	−0.007 (−0.25)
	The employed	−0.109*** (−4.61)	−0.587*** (−6.01)	−0.001 (−0.20)
Income level (reference group: low-income)	Lower-income	0.062** (2.49)	0.124 (0.99)	0.014** (2.28)
	Middle-income	0.105*** (3.62)	−0.007 (−0.05)	0.044*** (6.01)

(continued)

Table 13.2 (continued)

Variables		(1) Average length	(2) Average participants length	(3) Used or not
	Higher-income	0.139*** (4.53)	−0.005 (−0.04)	0.059*** (7.49)
	High-income	0.180*** (4.43)	0.106 (0.78)	0.064*** (6.17)
Constant term		0.772*** (3.38)	2.654*** (5.23)	0.248*** (5.58)
Observed value		24,053	5213	24,053
R^2		0.104	0.041	0.170
F value		101.6	7.859	246.4

Note T-values are in parentheses. ***, **, and * indicate that the estimated coefficients passed significance tests at the 1%, 5%, and 10% levels, respectively

Differences in Phone Reading Among Different Groups of People

In Fig. 13.6, the trends of phone reading usage rate of men and women of different ages were basically the same, with both reaching the peak at the age of 20–25. Comparing the two trends, women's reading usage rate was higher than men's before the age of 30, while men's reading usage rate was higher than women's after the age of 30.

In Fig. 13.7, it can be seen that the trends of reading usage rates of urban and rural residents of different ages were basically the same. Comparing the two trends, the reading usage rates of urban and rural residents were basically the same before the age of 20. After the age of 20, the phone reading usage rates of urban residents were significantly higher than those of rural residents. This may be due to the difference in

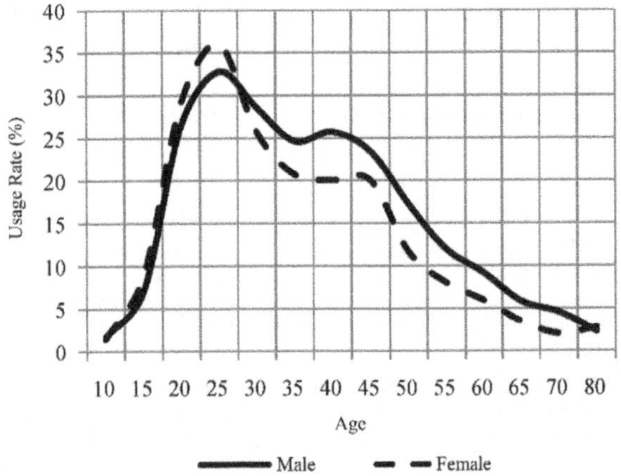

Fig. 13.6 Usage rate of phone reading by age and gender

the nature of work and lifestyle between urban and rural areas, where urban residents have a higher demand for information and knowledge than rural residents.

In Fig. 13.8, it can be seen that students had the highest usage rate of phone reading among the three groups of people. From the perspective of gender, the usage rate of phone reading was higher among female students and the unemployed than men, while among employed people, the usage rate was higher for men than women.

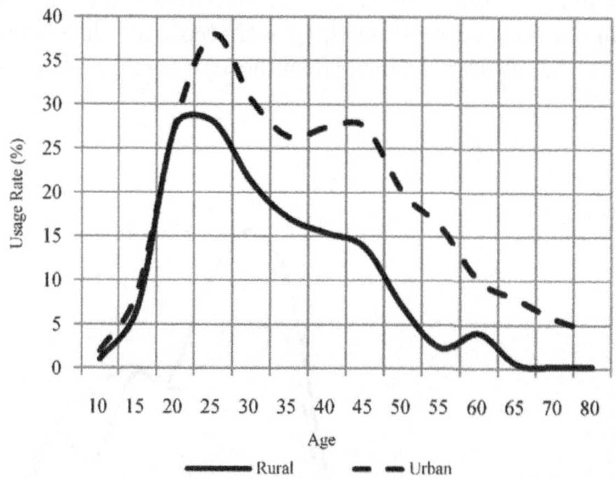

Fig. 13.7 Usage rate of phone reading by age and by urban and rural areas

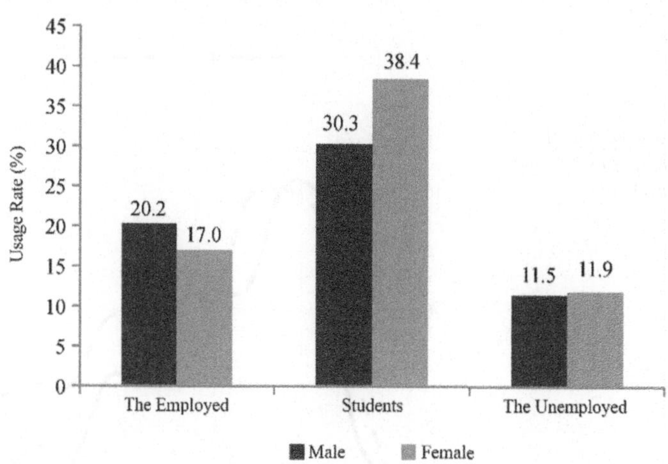

Fig. 13.8 Usage rate of phone reading by employment status and gender

Differences in Phone Socializing Among Different Groups of People

In Fig. 13.9, the trends of phone social use rates of men and women of different ages were basically the same. Comparing the two trends, the phone social usage rate of men was higher than that of women before the age of 40, while women's phone usage rate for socializing was higher than that of men after the age of 40.

In Fig. 13.10, the trends of usage rates of urban and rural residents of different ages were basically the same. Comparing the two trends, the usage rates of phone socializing among urban and rural residents were basically the same before the age of 20. In contrast, the rates were higher than those of rural residents after the age of 20.

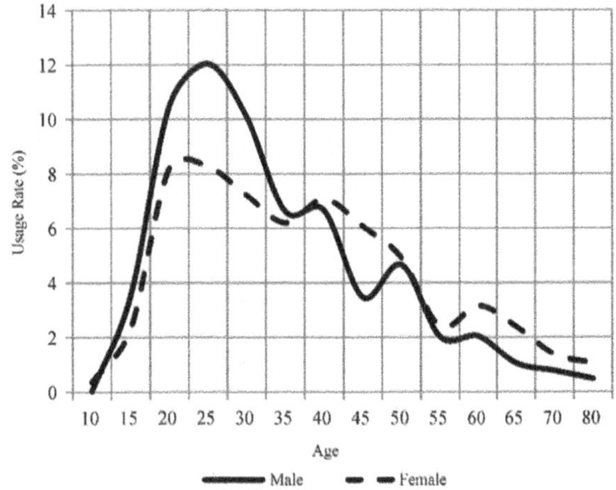

Fig. 13.9 Usage rate of phone socializing by age and gender

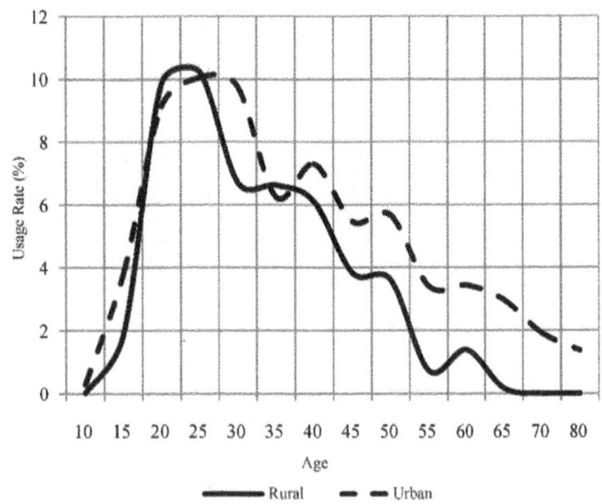

Fig. 13.10 Usage rate of phone socializing by age and urban and rural areas

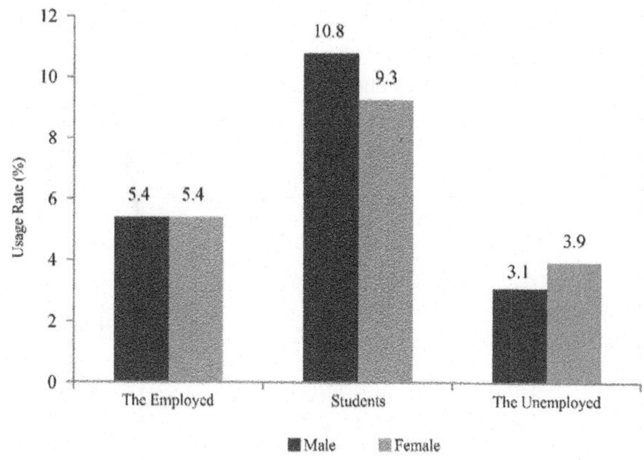

Fig. 13.11 Usage rate of phone socializing by employment status and gender

In Fig. 13.11, students had the highest usage rate of phone socializing among the three groups of people. From a gender perspective, the usage rate of phone socializing among male students was higher than that of women. For the employed, the usage rate was the same for both genders, but higher for women than men among the unemployed.

Differences in Watching and Listening on Phones

In Fig. 13.12, the trends of the usage rates of watching and listening on phones of men and women of different ages were basically the same. Comparing the two trends, before the age of 20, there was no difference in the usage rate between men and women, while from the age of 20, the usage rate of women was higher than that of men. After the age of 60, the usage rate between men and women was the same again.

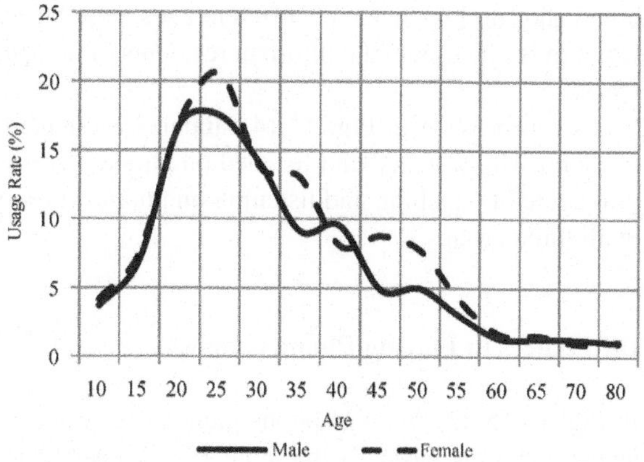

Fig. 13.12 Usage rate of watching and listening on phones by age and gender

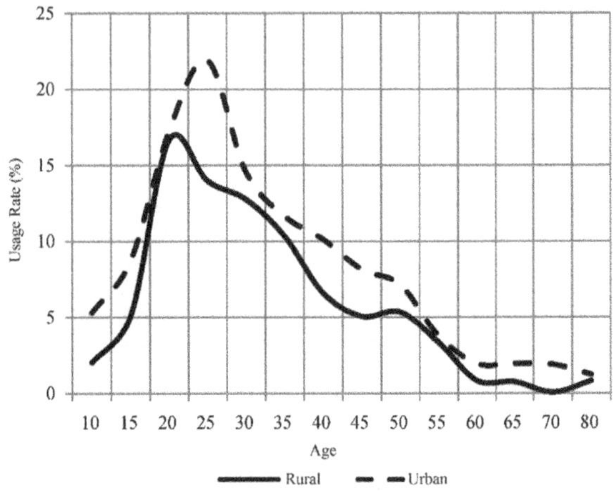

Fig. 13.13 Usage rate of watching and listening on phones by age and urban and rural areas

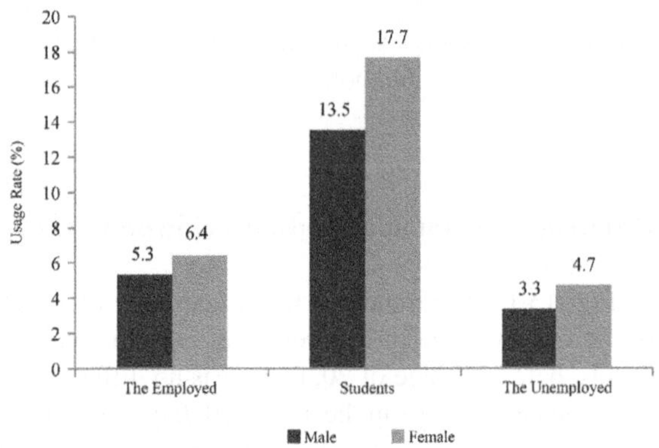

Fig. 13.14 Usage rate of watching and listening on phones by employment status and gender

From Fig. 13.13, the trend of usage rates of phone watching and listening for urban and rural residents of different ages were basically the same. Comparing the two trends, the usage rate of urban residents of all ages was higher than that of rural areas.

As can be seen in Fig. 13.14, students accounted for the largest proportion of residents who watched and listened on phones. From the perspective of gender, the usage rate of watching and listening on phones for women was higher than for men in all three groups.

Differences in Playing Phone Games

In Fig. 13.15, the trend of phone game usage rates of men and women in different age groups were basically the same, but the usage rate for men in all age groups was higher than that of women. Comparing it with the trend, it is possible that instead of watching videos and listening to music, men tended to play games.

In Fig. 13.16, it can be seen that the trends of phone game playing were basically the same for urban and rural residents in different age groups. Comparing the two trends, the usage rate was higher for urban residents than rural residents from 20 to 35 years old. After the age of 35, both urban and rural residents almost stopped using cell phones to play games.

In Fig. 13.17, it can be seen that the usage rate of playing games on phones was significantly higher for students than for the employed and the unemployed. Men used phones more for games than women.

In Fig. 13.18, it can be seen that the percentage of students using phones to play games was the highest for university students and above, reaching 38.8% and the

Fig. 13.15 Usage rate of phone games by age and gender

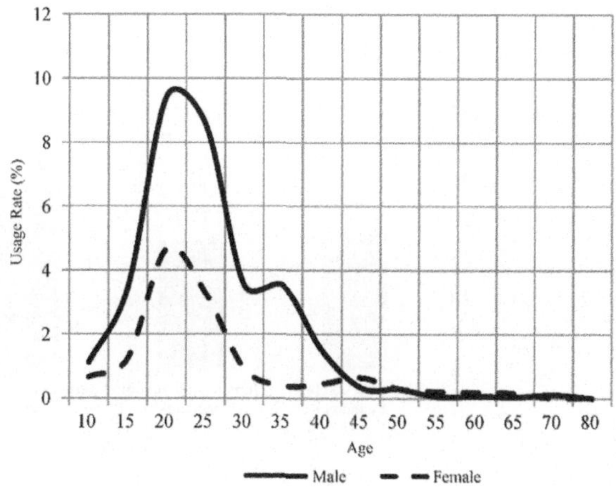

Fig. 13.16 Usage rate of phone games by age and urban and rural areas

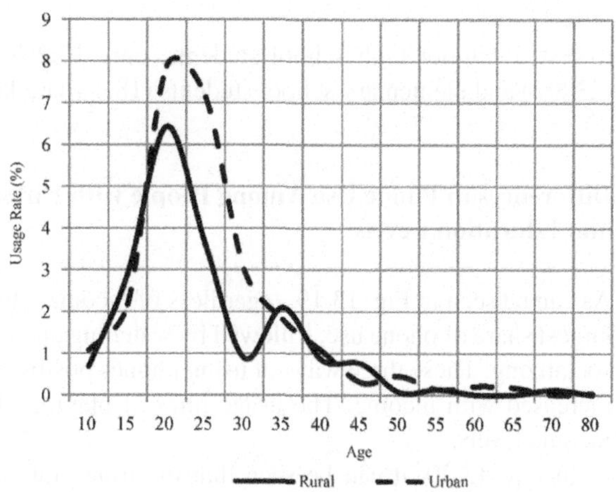

Fig. 13.17 Usage rate of playing games on phones by employment status and gender

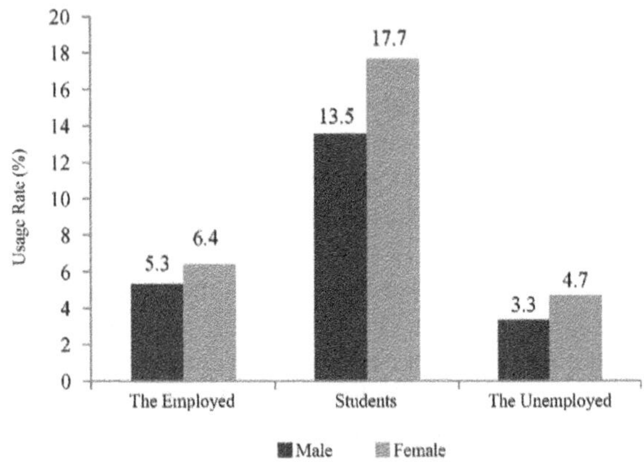

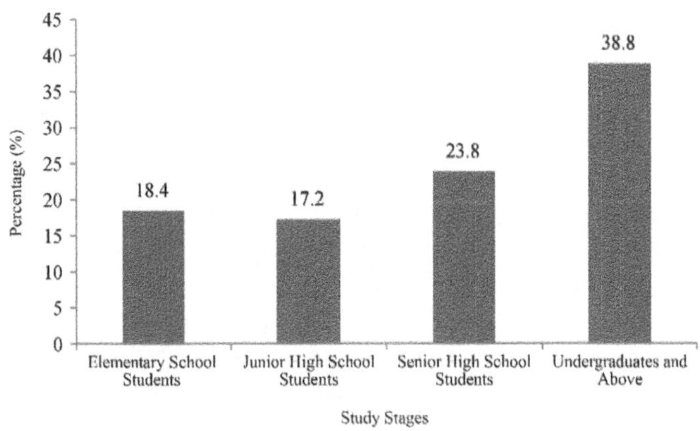

Fig. 13.18 Percentage of students playing games by study stage

lowest for junior high school students, only 17.2%. Senior high school students (23.8%) and elementary school students (18.4%) ranked second and third.

Differences in Phone Use Among People with Different Income and Education Levels

As can be seen in Fig. 13.19, regardless of income, phone reading accounted for the largest share of phone use, followed by watching and listening on phones, and phone socializing. These three ways of using phones positively correlated with income and increased with income. The usage rates of playing phone games were low for all income levels.

In Fig. 13.20, it can be seen that the usage rate of phones increased with the residents' education level. Residents who had not gone to school hardly used cell

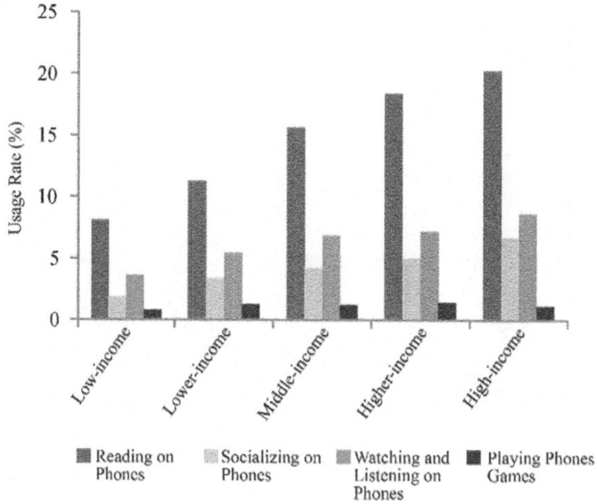

Fig. 13.19 Phone usage rate by income and use

phones, while residents with the education level of bachelor's or above have the highest usage rate of phones for all purposes. The usage rate of reading on phones was obviously higher than others with lower education levels.

As seen from Fig. 13.21, among the residents engaged in different occupations, the usage rate of phone reading was the highest among professional and technical staff, and the lowest among agriculture, forestry, animal husbandry and fishery production

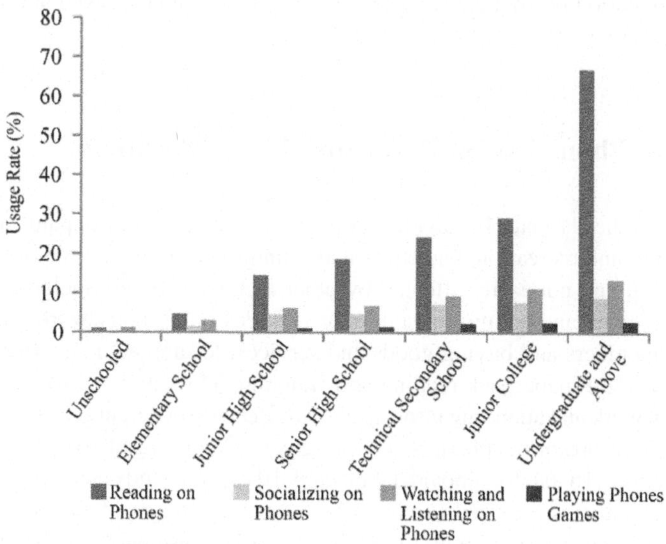

Fig. 13.20 Phone usage rate by education level and usage

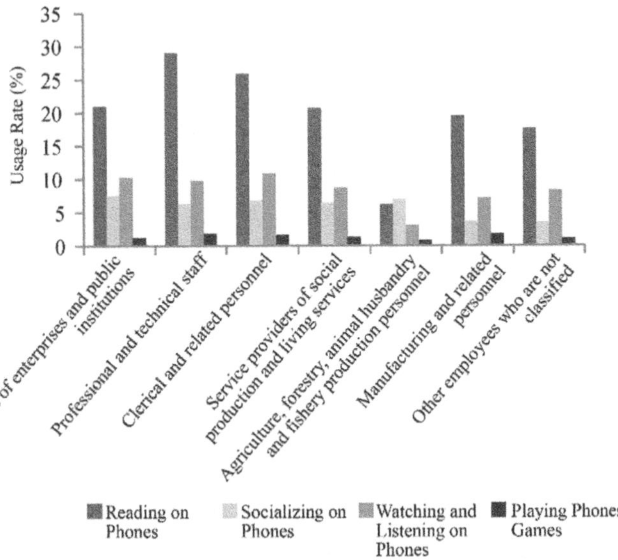

Fig. 13.21 Usage rate of phones by occupation and usage

personnel. Manufacturing and related personnel had the lowest usage rate of phone socializing, while people with other occupations had little difference in this regard. The highest usage rate for watching and listening on phones was among clerical personnel, and the lowest was among agricultural, forestry, animal husbandry and fishery production personnel. The usage rate of phone games stayed at a low level, not varying much among the occupational groups.

Impact of Phone Use on Residents' Time Allocation

The time of the day can be divided into five parts: self-care, unpaid labor, paid labor, leisure and recreation, and study and training, because the time of paid labor is more fixed and not easily affected by other factors. Self-care includes sleeping, personal hygiene and eating; unpaid labor includes doing housework, taking care of family members and buying goods and services; leisure and recreation includes physical exercise, paperback reading and watching TV; study and training include doing homework and attending tutoring classes. Because different activities are taken by different groups of people, this section selects samples aged 10–80 for self-care and recreation, 16–64 for unpaid labor, and 10–22 for study and training. First, descriptive statistics are used to compare the average hours of phone use among participants in each activity with residents who did not use phones. Then the extent and trends of the impact of phones on each activity were investigated by regressing the time spent on each activity on whether or not phones were used.

Table 13.3 shows that there are differences in the time allocation for each activity between residents who used phones and those who did not. Nationally and in urban and rural areas, residents who used phones spent less time sleeping, eating, doing housework, caring, doing physical exercise, doing paperback reading, and watching TV than those who did not. In contrast, residents who used phones spent more time on personal hygiene, buying goods and services, doing homework, and attending tutoring classes than those who did not use phones. This may be due, on the one hand, to the fact that those who did not use cell phones could use the time saved in other activities; on the other hand, it may also be due to group differences between those who used and did not use phones. Therefore, this study not only analyzes the effects of different individual characteristics on phone use, but also further analyzes the effects of phone use on time spent on other activities.

Since the time allocation among different activities is influenced not only by phone use but also by the individual characteristics of the owners, we use multiple regressions to analyze the impact of phones on other activities. The regression equation controlled for variables such as age, gender, urban and rural areas, education level, employment status and per capita household income. Strictly speaking, the regression results validate the correlation between phone use and other activities, but

Table 13.3 Average participants length in each activity. Unit: hours/day

Activity		Population					
		National total		Urban		Rural	
		Use phones	Not use	Use phones	Not use	Use phones	Not use
Self-care	Sleeping	8.38	8.42	8.36	8.39	8.44	8.46
	Personal hygiene activities	0.67	0.63	0.67	0.65	0.65	0.61
	Eating	1.58	1.68	1.58	1.67	1.57	1.68
Unpaid labor	Housework and caring	3.04	3.71	2.85	3.61	3.50	3.84
	Buying goods and services	1.77	1.75	1.77	1.63	1.79	2.11
Leisure and recreation	Physical exercise	1.79	2.22	1.84	2.26	1.60	2.13
	Paperback reading	1.69	1.90	1.83	2.01	1.20	1.56
	Watching TV	2.73	3.14	2.71	3.22	2.79	3.05
Study and training	Doing homework	2.95	2.62	2.98	2.89	2.91	2.18
	Attending tutoring classes	3.84	3.72	3.95	3.85	3.48	3.11

Table 13.4 Effect of phone use on time spent on each activity. Unit: hours/day

Activity		Results		
		Whether phones are used	T-value	Observed value
Self-care	Sleeping	−0.164***	−5.96	24,053
	Personal hygiene activities	0.069***	7.80	24,053
	Eating	−0.051***	−3.05	24,053
Unpaid labor	Housework and caring	−0.208***	−4.84	18,567
	Buying goods and services	0.045***	3.46	18,567
Leisure and recreation	Physical exercise	0.034	1.53	24,053
	Paperback reading	−0.016**	−2.05	24,053
	Watching TV	−0.356***	−10.03	24,053
Study and training	Doing homework	−0.284***	−3.40	3187
	Attending tutoring classes	−0.015	−0.44	3187

Note ***, **, and * indicate that the estimated coefficients passed the significance test at the 1%, 5%, and 10% levels, respectively

this is not causality, as phone use may be contemporaneously determined with other activities. The specific regression results are reported in Table 13.4.

From the regression results, residents who used cell phones slept 0.16 h per day less than those who did not, meaning that phone use crowded out some of the sleep time, a finding that was consistent with Demirci et al.,[5] who found that cell phone use reduced sleep time and sleep quality among students. The regression results for personal hygiene and eating showed that similarly, phone use reduced time for eating and increased time for personal hygiene. Why does cell phone use increase personal hygiene time? This may be due to the following two reasons: first, phone users are more aware of the requirements and changes in society, and thus will have higher requirements for personal image, so they will spend more time on personal hygiene activities, such as dressing, makeup, beauty, hairdressing, etc.; second, when performing personal hygiene activities, such as washing and toileting, if they also use phones to listen to news or watch videos, they may increase the personal hygiene time required for the activity.

Phone use crowds out time spent doing housework and caring for family members by an average of 0.21 h per day, which is in line with the same conclusion reached by Wallsten.[6] The residents who use phones also spend more time buying goods and

[5] Demirci K, Akgnül M. Akpinar A. "Relationship of Smartphone Use Severity with Sleep Quality, Depression, and Anxiety in University Students", *Journal of Behavior Addictions*, 2015, 4 (2).

[6] Wallsten S., "What are We Not Doing When We're Online?", *Social Science Electronic Publishing*, 2013.

services, which may be due to the more convenient online shopping used by residents with more shopping needs.

There is no significant effect of phone use on time spent on physical exercise, which may be related to the fact that modern people are becoming more health conscious. However, the use of cell phones has crowded out the time for paper reading. Jiang Xiaoyuan[7] believes that the fundamental confrontation between electronic reading and paperback reading lies in "fragmented reading". The increase in phone reading is due to its portability. People can read at any fragmented time. Moreover, with the development of the Internet, the amount of information available from cell phones is increasing, which is the most important reason why paperback reading cannot be reached in today's fast-paced life.

As we can see from Table 13.4, the use of phones also crowds out the time for watching TV. Jiyoung Cha[8] believes that the media substitution theory, based on the Principle of Relative Constant or Zero-Sum Game, is that residents' attention resources and advertisers' input resources are limited and relatively constant. The emergence of new media will divert resources from existing media, thus forming a zero-sum competition among media. Ferguson[9] argues that whether a new medium can replace an existing one depends on whether it can functionally satisfy the needs of residents better than the existing one. It is obvious that cell phones are so rich in functions that they can replace the functions of TV. The portability of cell phones has shifted the "living room culture" to the "bedroom culture".

There is a negative correlation between using cell phones and students' time spent doing homework. Students who used cell phones spent 0.28 h per day less time doing homework than those who did not use cell phones. There is no significant effect on the time spent attending tutoring classes, probably because attending tutorial classes is a mandatory requirement for parents rather than something students can decide on their own.

In Fig. 13.22, it can be seen that the sleep time of those who use cell phones under the age of 20 was higher than that of those who did not use cell phones. In contrast, the sleep time of those who used cell phones after the age of 20 was lower than that of those who did not use cell phones.

As can be seen in Fig. 13.23, the time spent on housework and care-giving was higher for non-phone users than for phone users at any age. Looking at the trend of the change in time spent on household care-giving, a peak was reached around 30, which is related to the fact that most Chinese residents in this age group have their first child. As the child ages, the time spent involved in care-giving begins to decline, dropping to a low point around the age of 50, and then bouncing back, which may be due to the birth of grandchildren in families in this age group.

[7] Xiaoyuan Jiang, "The Future of Reading: An Optimistic Outlook—On E-Reading and Paper Reading", *Editors Monthly*, 2013 (3).

[8] Jiyoung Cha, "Do Online Video Platforms Cannibalize Television? How Viewers are Moving from Old Screens to New Ones", *Journal of Advertising Research*, 2013, 53 (1).

[9] Ferguson, Douglas A. and Perse, Elizabeth M., "The World Wide Web as a Functional Alternative to Television", *Journal of Broadcasting & Electronic Media*, 2000, 44 (2).

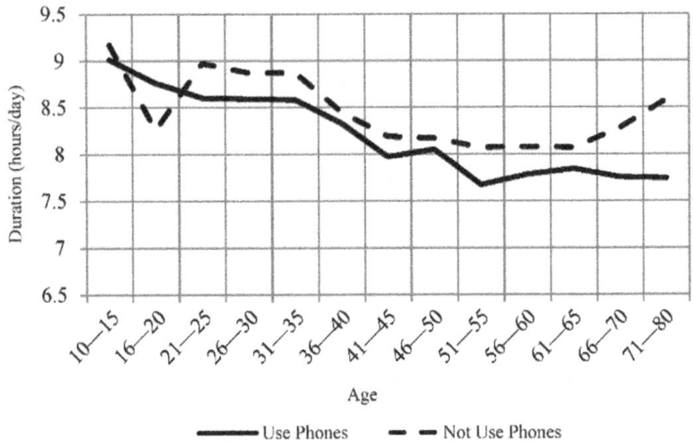

Fig. 13.22 Comparison of sleep time by age and groups

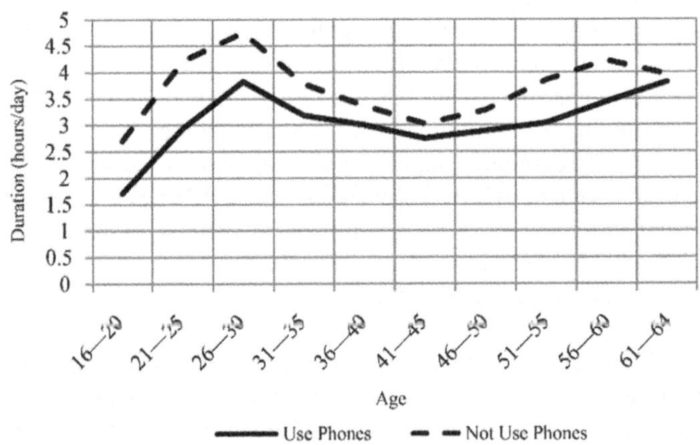

Fig. 13.23 Comparison of housework and care time by age and groups

As seen in Fig. 13.24, residents who used cell phones before the age of 20 read paper books for a longer period. In general, after the age of 20, it was those who did not use mobile phones after age 20 spent more time reading printed books than those who did.

Figure 13.25 shows that in almost all age groups, those who did not use cell phones spent more time watching TV than those who used cell phones. From the variation trend, the viewing time of both groups is in a U-shape, with the lowest point of the cell phone crowd appearing at 31–35 years old and the lowest point of the non-cell phone crowd appearing at 36–40 years old.

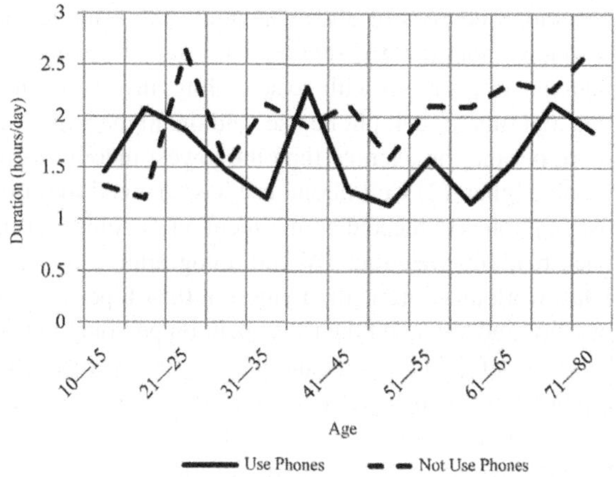

Fig. 13.24 Comparison of reading time of paperback books by age and groups

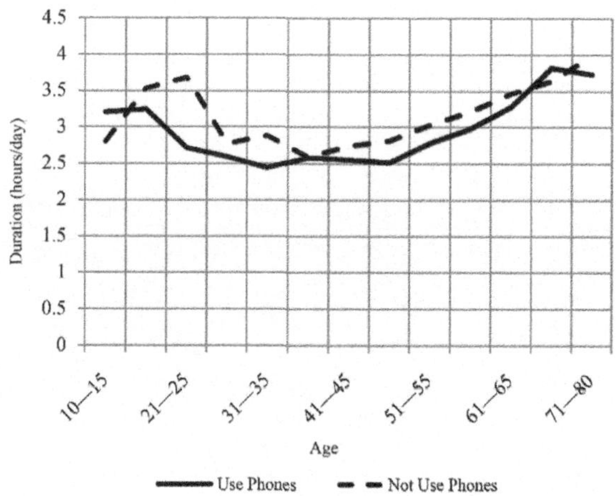

Fig. 13.25 Comparison of TV viewing time by age and population

Summary

Cell phones are an essential carrier of information in modern society and have influenced every aspect of residents' daily lives. This chapter uses data from the 2017 Chinese Time Use Survey to analyze the profile of phone use among Chinese residents, the differences in phone use among different groups, and the impact of phone use on time allocation for daily activities. The main conclusions are as follows. (1) There are differences in phone use among different groups, i.e., the digital divide. After controlling for other factors, cell phone use in urban areas is significantly higher than that in rural areas, with the former being about 6% points higher than the latter and the average length of time being about 0.1 h per day; the average length of time spent on phone use by residents aged 19–22 is higher than that of other age groups. There is a positive correlation between education and usage rate, with those with bachelor's degrees or above spending 0.5 h longer on average per day than those who have not attended school. The usage rate of cell phones is 19% points higher than that of residents with no schooling; income is directly proportional to the usage rate and time of cell phone use, and the highest quintile income earners spend 0.2 h more per day on average than the lowest income earners, and the usage rate is 6% points higher. (2) Cell phone use has changed the time allocation of residents. The use of phones reduced the time spent on sleeping, eating, housework and care, paperback reading, watching TV and doing homework, among which the time spent on housework and care is the longest at 0.21 h per day, followed by sleeping at 0.16 h per day, and extended the time spent on personal hygiene and purchasing goods and services at 0.07 h per day and 0.05 h per day, respectively. There was no significant effect on physical exercise and tutoring time. Overall, cell phone use can bring more information and convenience to people, but it can also crowd out sleep or leisure time and reduce people's quality of life.